Frailty and Kidney Disease

AF883484

Carlos Guido Musso • José Ricardo Jauregui
Juan Florencio Macías-Núñez • Adrian Covic
Editors

Frailty and Kidney Disease

A Practical Guide to Clinical Management

Springer

Editors
Carlos Guido Musso
Hospital Italiano de Buenos Aires
Buenos Aires
Argentina

José Ricardo Jauregui
Hospital Italiano de Buenos Aires
Buenos Aires
Argentina

Juan Florencio Macías-Núñez
University of Salamanca
Salamanca
Spain

Adrian Covic
Grigore T. Popa University of Medicine
Iasi
Romania

ISBN 978-3-030-53528-5 ISBN 978-3-030-53529-2 (eBook)
https://doi.org/10.1007/978-3-030-53529-2

© Springer Nature Switzerland AG 2021
This work is subject to copyright. All rights are reserved by the Publisher, whether the whole or part of the material is concerned, specifically the rights of translation, reprinting, reuse of illustrations, recitation, broadcasting, reproduction on microfilms or in any other physical way, and transmission or information storage and retrieval, electronic adaptation, computer software, or by similar or dissimilar methodology now known or hereafter developed.
The use of general descriptive names, registered names, trademarks, service marks, etc. in this publication does not imply, even in the absence of a specific statement, that such names are exempt from the relevant protective laws and regulations and therefore free for general use.
The publisher, the authors and the editors are safe to assume that the advice and information in this book are believed to be true and accurate at the date of publication. Neither the publisher nor the authors or the editors give a warranty, expressed or implied, with respect to the material contained herein or for any errors or omissions that may have been made. The publisher remains neutral with regard to jurisdictional claims in published maps and institutional affiliations.

This Springer imprint is published by the registered company Springer Nature Switzerland AG
The registered company address is: Gewerbestrasse 11, 6330 Cham, Switzerland

To our family and patients

Foreword

Frailty is a geriatric syndrome, not a specific disease, that is defined by a number of clinical manifestations, including unintentional weight loss, declining strength, and low physical activity. It can be recognized by application of several well-established and validated scoring systems. It is common among the elderly and very elderly, and accounts for substantial morbidity and mortality, especially due to falls and delayed recovery from inter-current illnesses. Frailty is a dynamic process, and at the individual level, its status can change dramatically over time. Pathophysiologically, muscle loss (sarcopenia) and bone fragility (osteopenia) contribute greatly to the origins of the syndrome.

While frailty has received great attention in the geriatric literature, it has received only scanty and superficial scrutiny by the discipline of nephrology. This deficiency has now been corrected by Carlos G. Musso, MD, PhD, and his collaborators by the publication of this treatise dedicated to the subject of frailty and kidney disease. The 14 chapters, each lucidly written by an expert in the field, provide broad coverage concerning the impact of frailty in chronic and acute kidney disease, dialysis, and transplantation. Many "pearls of wisdom" will be encountered during a thorough reading of the text and such moments will undoubtedly contribute to improved management of this often-neglected syndrome in patients with renal disease.

As chronicled by Shakespeare in *As You Like It*—the "sixth age of the lean and slipper'd pantallon and the shrunk shank" can now be modified by the insertion of the "dwindling kidneys." The *Frailty and Kidney Disease* monograph is a timely and welcome addition to the literature of nephrology. It does not disappoint.

Richard J. Glassock, MD, MACP, FASN
Geffen School of Medicine at UCLA
Laguna Niguel, CA, USA
December 26, 2019

Preface

Frailty is a condition not merely induced by ageing, but mainly due to a progressive and sustained deterioration in the functional reserve of skeletal muscle; nervous, endocrine, and immune systems; as well as poor coordination among them. This phenomenon leads to an altered homeostatic response, and consequently to an increased vulnerability towards stressors.

Frailty prevalence increases steadily with age from 4% in older individuals to 26% in the oldest old. In this age group, frailty status is tightly related to the geriatric syndromes: delirium, incontinence, gait disorders, falls, and immobility syndrome. These are also known as "geriatric giants" due to their high prevalence and great impact on geriatric health.

Any form of kidney disease, acute, chronic, or on replacement therapy, constitutes a serious condition and its prevalence also increases with age. Moreover, its association with frailty leads to a diverse condition (senescent nephropathy) that has worse evolution and prognosis.

In the present book, the state of the art of frailty status and its impact on geriatric syndromes as well as the entire spectrum of kidney disease are deeply analyzed with the intention of providing a useful guide to daily medical activity.

Buenos Aires, Argentina — Carlos Guido Musso
Buenos Aires, Argentina — José Ricardo Jauregui
Salamanca, Spain — Juan Florencio Macías-Núñez
Iasi, Romania — Adrian Covic

Contents

Contributors

Gustavo Aroca-Martinez, MD, PhD Facultad de Ciencias de la Salud, Universidad Simon Bolivar, Barranquilla, Colombia

Nephrology Division, Clinica de la Costa, Barranquilla, Colombia

Angela Benjumea, MD Faculty of Health Sciences, Caldas University, Caldas, Colombia

Maria Valeria Beruto, MD Clinical Pharmacology Section, Hospital Italiano de Buenos Aires, Buenos Aires, Argentina

Olivia M. Capalbo Physiology Department, Instituto Universitario de Buenos Aires, Buenos Aires, Argentina

Malena Colombo Physiology Department, Instituto Universitario del Hospital Italiano de Buenos Aires, Buenos Aires, Argentina

Candela Conti Physiology Department, Instituto Universitario del Hospital Italiano de Buenos Aires, Buenos Aires, Argentina

Adrian Covic, PhD, FERA, FRCP, FESC University of Medicine and Pharmacy Grigore T. Popa, Iasi, Romania

Nephrology Division, Dr.C.I. Parhon Hospital, Iasi, Romania

María del Pilar Romero Physiology Department, Instituto Universitario del Hospital Italiano de Buenos Aires, Buenos Aires, Argentina

Gustavo Duque, MD, PhD, FRACP, FGSA Australian Institute for Musculoskeletal Science (AIMSS), The University of Melbourne and Western Health, St. Albans, VIC, Australia

Department of Medicine-Western Health, The University of Melbourne, St. Albans, VIC, Australia

Gabriel Echeverri, MD Clinica de la Costa, Barranquilla, Colombia

Elbio Mariano Esperatti, MD, PhD Hospital Privado de Comunidad, Mar del Plata, Argentina

Escuela Superior de Medicina, Universidad Nacional de Mar del Plata, Mar del Plata, Argentina

Jack Feehan, BSc (Clin Sci), MH Sc (Osteo) Australian Institute for Musculoskeletal Science (AIMSS), The University of Melbourne and Western Health, St. Albans, VIC, Australia

Department of Medicine-Western Health, The University of Melbourne, St. Albans, VIC, Australia

Carlos Lautaro Franco Physiology Department, Instituto Universitario del Hospital Italiano de Buenos Aires, Buenos Aires, Argentina

Nora Angélica Fuentes, MD Hospital Privado de Comunidad, Mar del Plata, Argentina

Escuela Superior de Medicina, Universidad Nacional de Mar del Plata, Mar del Plata, Argentina

Angel Golimstok, MD Cognition and Behaviour Section, Department of Neurology, Hospital Italiano Buenos Aires, Buenos Aires, Argentina

María Eugenia González, MD Hospital Privado de Comunidad, Mar del Plata, Argentina

Escuela Superior de Medicina, Universidad Nacional de Mar del Plata, Mar del Plata, Argentina

Henry González-Torres, MSc Facultad de Ciencias de la Salud, Universidad Simon Bolivar, Barranquilla, Colombia

Universidad del Valle, Cali, Colombia

Kristian Heldal, MD, PhD, MHA Department of Transplantation Medicine, Section of Nephrology, Oslo University Hospital, Oslo, Norway

Adina Carmen Ilie, MD, PhD University of Medicine and Pharmacy Grigore T. Popa, Iasi, Romania

Division of Geriatric Medicine & Gerontology, Dr.C.I. Parhon Hospital, Iasi, Romania

José Ricardo Jauregui, MD, PhD Hospital Italiano de Buenos Aires, Buenos Aires, Argentina

University of Buenos Aires, Buenos Aires, Argentina

Mateo Lombardi Physiology Department, Instituto Universitario del Hospital Italiano de Buenos Aires, Buenos Aires, Argentina

Cynthia Irene Mariñansky, MD Geriatric Division, Durand Hospital, Buenos Aires, Argentina

Maimonides University, Buenos Aires, Argentina

Tahir Masud, MBBS, MA, MSc, FRCP Nottingham University Hospitals NHS Trust, Nottingham, UK

Victor Gastón Moreno-Milicich, MD Cognition and Behaviour Section, Department of Neurology, Hospital Italiano Buenos Aires, Buenos Aires, Argentina

Manuel Montero-Odasso, MD, PhD, AGSF, FGSA, FRCPC Departments of Medicine, and Epidemiology and Biostatistics, The University of Western Ontario, London, ON, Canada

Division of Geriatric Medicine, Parkwood Institute, The University of Western Ontario, London, ON, Canada

Lawson Health Research Institute, London, ON, Canada

Gait and Brain Lab, Parkwood Institute, London, ON, Canada

Carlos G. Musso, MD, PhD Physiology Department, Instituto Universitario del Hospital Italiano de Buenos Aires, Buenos Aires, Argentina

Facultad de Ciencias de la Salud, Universidad Simon Bolivar, Barranquilla, Colombia

Nephrology Division, Hospital Italiano de Buenos Aires, Buenos Aires, Argentina

Ageing Biology Unit, Hospital Italiano de Buenos Aires, Buenos Aires, Argentina

Guido M. Musso-Enz Facultad de Medicina, Universidad Católica Argentina, Buenos Aires, Argentina

Victoria P. Musso-Enz Physiology Department, Instituto Universitario del Hospital Italiano de Buenos Aires, Buenos Aires, Argentina

Dana M. Mysler Physiology Department, Instituto Universitario del Hospital Italiano de Buenos Aires, Buenos Aires, Argentina

Andra Nastasa, MD University of Medicine and Pharmacy Grigore T. Popa, Iasi, Romania

Nephrology Division, Dr.C. I. Parhon Hospital, Iasi, Romania

Steven Phu, MSc Department of Medicine-Western Health, The University of Melbourne, St. Albans, VIC, Australia

Falls, Balance and Injury Research Centre, Neuroscience Research Australia, University of New South Wales, Sydney, NSW, Australia

Nadia E. Savoy, MD Clinical Pharmacology Section, Hospital Italiano de Buenos Aires, Buenos Aires, Argentina

Paula Scibona, MD Clinical Pharmacology Section, Hospital Italiano de Buenos Aires, Buenos Aires, Argentina

Ventura A. Simonovich, MD Clinical Pharmacology Section, Hospital Italiano de Buenos Aires, Buenos Aires, Argentina

Carlos Zuniga-San Martin, MD, MSc Facultad de Medicina, Universidad Catolica de la Santisima Concepcion, Bio Bio, Chile

Facultad de Medicina, Universidad de Concepcion, Bio Bio, Chile

Instituto de Nefrologia Concepcion, Bio Bio, Chile

Chapter 1
Frailty Phenotype

Angela Benjumea

A frailty consensus in 2012 defined frailty as follows: "A medical syndrome with multiple causes and contributors that is characterized by diminished strength, endurance, and reduced physiologic function that increases an individual's vulnerability for developing increased dependency and/or death" [1]. In addition, frailty is considered a clinical syndrome, with increased vulnerability, and susceptibility to minimal stress, which can cause functional impairment. Frailty, can be reversible or at least attenuated by interventions, and its early detection is highly useful in primary and community care [1].

Frailty is either physical or psychological, or a combination of the two components, and is a dynamic condition that can improve or worsen over time. Two approaches in defining physical frailty have become popular [1]. The deficit model consists of adding together an individual's number of impairments and conditions to create a Frailty Index [2]. The second model originally defined a specific physical phenotype consisting of a constellation of five possible components such as weight loss, exhaustion, weakness, slowness, and reduced physical activity. From this perspective, pre-frail (one or two components), and frail status ($\geq$3 components) represent different degrees of an underlying physiologic state of multisystemic and energetic dysregulation [3].

Both of these definitions are currently used to define a frail and a pre-frail state (a condition between frail and non-frail). Frailty domains appear to belong to a common construct, with physical strength being one of the discriminating characteristics [4]. Numerous other frailty definitions have been developed, most of them based on one of the other basic approaches. Simple rapid screening tests have been developed and validated to allow physicians to rapidly recognize frail people. Examples of some commonly used and validated frailty tools include the FRAIL,

A. Benjumea (✉)
Faculty of Health Sciences, Caldas University, Caldas, Colombia
e-mail: angela.benjumea@ucaldas.edu.co

© Springer Nature Switzerland AG 2021

C. G. Musso et al. (eds.), *Frailty and Kidney Disease*,
https://doi.org/10.1007/978-3-030-53529-2_1

the Cardiovascular Health Study Frailty Screening Measure, the Clinical Frailty Scale, and the Gerontopole Frailty Screening Tool. It is accepted that such instruments can be used to identify frail subjects who need assessment [1].

Since 2001, Fried et al. described that the prevalence of frailty increases with age, confering a high risk of adverse health outcomes such as mortality, institutionalization, falls, and hospitalization. Numerous geriatric interventions have been developed to improve clinical outcomes for frail older adults. A major obstacle to the success of such interventions has been the absence of a standardized and valid screening method for those who are truly frail in order to effectively decide the patient's target care. At that time, there was a growing consensus that frailty markers include age-associated declines in lean body mass, strength, endurance, balance, walking performance, and low activity, and that multiple components must be present clinically to constitute frailty. Many of these factors are related, and can be theoretically unified into a cycle of frailty. From this perspective, frailty is conceptualized as a syndrome of decreased resiliency and reserves, in which a mutually exacerbating cycle of declines across multiple systems results in negative energy balance, sarcopenia, and diminished strength and tolerance to exertion. This being associated with a declined body energy and reserve. The core elements of this cycle are those commonly identified as clinical signs and symptoms of frailty. Then, Fried et al. evaluated whether this phenotype could identify high risk patients to present adverse health outcomes [3].

This study employed data from the Cardiovascular Health Study (CHS), a prospective, observational study of men and women 65 years and older. The original cohort (*N:* 5201) was recruited from four US communities in 1989–90. An additional cohort of 687 African American men and women was recruited in 1992–93 from three cities.

They were operationalized utilizing data collected in CHS, specifying that a phenotype of frailty was identified by the presence of three or more of the following components of the hypothesized cycle of frailty [3].

The criteria used to define frailty were the following:

- *Weight loss*: In this criteria the evaluating question is: "Have you lost more than 10 pounds unintentionally in the last year (i.e., not due to dieting or exercise)?" If the answer is "yes", then weight loss is considered as a frail criterion. If this were to be evaluated during follow-up, weight loss is calculated as follows: (Weight in previous year – current measured weight)/(weight in previous year) = K. If $K \geq 0.05$, and the subject does not report that he/she was trying to lose weight (i.e., unintentional weight loss of at least 5% of previous year's body weight), then weight loss = Yes.
- *Exhaustion*: In this criteria CES–D Depression Scale is used, and the following two statements are read. (a) I felt that everything I did required an effort. (b) I could not get going. The following question is asked: "How often in the last week did you feel this way?" 0 = rarely or none of the time (1 day), 1 = some or a little of the time (1–2 days), 2 = a moderate amount of the time (3–4 days), or 3 = most of the time. Subjects answering "2" or "3" to either of these questions are categorized as frail by the exhaustion criterion.

- *Physical Activity*: This criteria is based on the short version of the Minnesota Leisure Time Activity questionnaire, asking about walking, chores (moderately strenuous), mowing the lawn, raking, gardening, hiking, jogging, biking, exercise cycling, dancing, aerobics, bowling, golf, singles tennis, doubles tennis, racquetball, calisthenics, swimming. Here, expended Kcals per week are calculated using standardized algorithm,and this variable is stratified by gender.
  Men: Those with 383 Kcals of physical activity per week are frail.
  Women: Those with 270 Kcals per week are frail.
- *Walk Time*: Stratified by gender and height

Men	*Cutoff for Time to Walk 15 feet criterion for frailty*
Height ≤173 cm	≥7 seconds
Height >173 cm	≥6 seconds
Women	
Height ≤159 cm	≥7 seconds
Height >159 cm	≥6 seconds

- *Grip Strength*: Stratified by gender and body mass index (BMI) quartiles:

Men	*Cutoff for grip strength (Kg) criterion for frailty*
BMI ≤24	≤29
BMI 24.1–26	≤30
BMI 26.1–28	≤30
BMI >28	≤32
Women	
BMI ≤23	≤17
BMI 23.1–26	≤17.3
BMI 26.1–29	≤18
BMI >29	≤21

In summary, the criteria were as follows:

1. Shrinking: weight loss, unintentional, of ≥10 pounds in prior year or, at follow-up, of ≥5% of body weight in prior year (by direct measurement of weight).
2. Weakness: grip strength in the lowest 20% at baseline, adjusted for gender and body mass index.
3. Poor endurance and energy: as indicated by self-report exhaustion. Self-reported exhaustion, identified by two questions from the CES–D scale [5], is associated with stage of exercise reached in graded exercise testing, as an indicator of VO2 max [6], and is predictive of cardiovascular disease [7].
4. Slowness: the slowest 20% of the population was defined at baseline, based on time to walk 15 feet, adjusting for gender and standing height.
5. Low physical activity level: A weighted score of kilocalories expended per week was calculated at baseline [8, 9], based on each participant's report. The lowest quintile of physical activity was identified for each gender.

For measures that identified the lowest quintile, the level established at baseline was applied to follow-up evaluations. A critical number of characteristics, defined as three or more, had to be present for an individual to be considered frail. Those with no characteristics were considered robust, whereas those with one or two characteristics were hypothesized to be in an intermediate, possibly pre-frail stage clinically [3].

The 5317 people evaluated were 65–101 years of age, 58% were female and 15% African American, with a broad range of socioeconomic, functional, and health status data. Those who were frail were older, more likely to be female and African American, and had less education, lower income, poorer health, and higher rates of comorbid chronic diseases and disability than those who were neither in the frail nor in the intermediate group. The frail group also had significantly higher rates of cardiovascular and pulmonary diseases, arthritis, and diabetes mellitus. However, there was no significant difference in the cancer rates, possibly due to the fact that the recruitment criteria excluded those under cancer treatment . Notably, 7% of those who were frail had none of mentioned chronic diseases, and 25% had just one. Among these diseases were: 56% arthritis, 25% hypertension, 8% diabetes mellitus, and less than 5% angina, congestive heart failure, cancer, and pulmonary disease. Both lower cognition and greater depressive symptoms were associated with frailty, and further showed an association between this phenotype and self-reported physical disability determined by the *instrumental activities of daily living* (IADLs) and the *activities of daily living* (ADLs). The above mentioned, displays the overlap and interrelation between these domains; frailty is distinct from, but overlaps with, both comorbidity (defined as a two or more chronic diseases or conditions) and disability (physical or mental impairment that substantially limits one or more of the major life activities). In addition, both frailty and comorbidity predict disability: disability may exacerbate frailty and comorbidity, and comorbid diseases may contribute, at least additively, to the development of frailty. An individual can experience, simultaneously, multiple symptoms of comorbid diseases, difficulty in ADLs, and the progressive weakness and vulnerability associated with frailty. The causal interconnectedness of these conditions, as well as their co-occurrence, makes their diagnosis and treatment key to improving overall health outcomes for older adults. Clinical outcomes for these patients will likely benefit from improving our ability to differentiate these entities and target therapies [10].

To assess whether three criteria predicted mortality significantly better than two, the predictive power of each combination of three criteria were compared. The results showed that, groups with three positive frailty components had a significantly worse survival rate than those with only two components, or without frailty. Based on these models, it was concluded that criteria based on three components, provided improved predictive power in identifying mortality risk. This work proposed a standardized phenotype of frailty in older adults and showed predictive validity for the adverse outcomes that geriatricians identified that frail older adults were at risk for: falls, hospitalizations, disability, and death. Even after adjusting measures of socioeconomic status, health status, subclinical and clinical disease, depressive symptoms, and disability status at baseline, frailty remained an independent predictor of risk of these adverse outcomes. The intermediate group with one or two frailty characteristics was at elevated, but still intermediate, risk for the above mentioned outcomes, and subsequent frailty.

This study provided insight into frailty and its outcomes in an older adult population who were neither institutionalized nor terminal patients. A standardized frailty phenotype provides the basis for future comparison with other populations [3].

The phenotype proposed by Fried offers greater predictive validity, compared with using only two criteria, and frailty charcaterization provided new insights into potential etiologies where aging and chronic illness constitute a final common pathways. The definition of frailty offered a validated and standardized, physiologically based definition applicable to the spectrum of frailty presentations seen in community-dwelling older adults. These frailty diagnosing criteria have been relatively easy and inexpensive to apply, and have offered the basis for standardized screening for frailty and risk of frailty in older adults. Frailty phenotype has been used to establish clinical risk of adverse outcomes.

In 2006, one study [11] evaluated the cross-validity, criterion validity, and internal validity in the Women's Health and Aging Studies (WHAS) of a discrete measure of frailty validated in the Cardiovascular Health Study (CHS). In the results, the frailty distributions in the WHAS and CHS were comparable. In proportional hazards models, frail women had a higher risk of developing ADL and/or instrumental ADL disability, institutionalization, and death, independently of multiple potentially confounding factors. The findings of this study were consistent with the widely held theory that conceptualizes frailty as a syndrome and states that the frailty definition developed in the CHS is applicable across diverse population samples and identifies a profile of high risk of multiple adverse outcomes.

Since 2001, more than 27 frailty measuring tools and/or definitions which aimed to diagnose the syndrome have been published. The frailty phenotype by Fried and colleagues (the Cardiovascular Health Study Index [CHS]) and the Frailty Index (FI) by Mitnitski and colleagues had their validity assessed in more than three different samples and are the two most frequently used strategies for frailty diagnosis (69% and 12% of published studies, respectively) [12]. However, both the CHS phenotype and the FI are difficult to put into practice in clinical or large epidemiological settings. The former requires objective measures implemented by trained staff and the latter a clinical database with information regarding different signs, symptoms, and health problems. Considering the reality of developing nations, with several professional and structural deficiencies in the health care system, simple frailty screening instruments present greater adequacy to service demands. The use of more complex instruments should be reserved for specialized geriatric services. Therefore, alternative frailty assessments, relying mostly on self-reported measures, have been recommended to a broad clinical context. Critically, the other tools have not had their diagnostic accuracy compared with commonly accepted frailty criteria such as the CHS phenotype criteria, and the use of these frailty evaluating tools depends on the clinical scenario.

References

1. Morley JE, Vellas B, et al. Frailty consensus: a call to action. J Am Med Dir Assoc. 2013;14(6):392–7. https://doi.org/10.1016/j.jamda.2013.03.022.
2. Mitnitski AB, Mogilner AJ, Rockwood K. Accumulation of deficits as a proxy measure of aging. Sci World J. 2001;1:323e336.
3. Fried LP, Tangen CM, Walston J, Cardiovascular Health Study Collaborative Research Group, et al. Frailty in older adults: evidence for a phenotype. J Gerontol A Biol Sci Med Sci. 2001;56:M146eM156.
4. Sourial N, Bergman H, Karunananthan S, et al. Contribution of frailty markers in explaining differences among individuals in five samples of older persons. J Gerontol A Biol Sci Med Sci. 2012;67:1197–204. [PubMed: 22459619]).
5. Orme J, Reis J, Herz E. Factorial and discriminate validity of the Center for Epidemiological Studies depression (CES-D) scale. J Clin Psychol. 1986;42:28–33.
6. Kop WJ, Appels APWM, Mendes de Leon CF, et al. The relationship between severity of coronary artery disease and vital exhaustion. J Psychosom Res. 1996;40:397–405.
7. Kop WJ, Appels APWM, Mendes de Leon CF, et al. Vital exhaustion predicts new cardiac events after successful coronary angioplasty. Psychosom Med. 1994;56:281–7.
8. Taylor HL, Jacobs DR, Schuker B, et al. A questionnaire for the assessment of leisure-time physical activities. J Chronic Dis. 1978;31:745–55.
9. Siscovick DS, Fried LP, Mittelmark M, for the Cardiovascular Health Study Research Group, et al. Exercise and subclinical cardiovascular disease in the elderly: the Cardiovascular Health Study. Am J Epidemiol. 1997;145:977–86.
10. Fried LP, Ferrucci L, Darer J, et al. Untangling the concepts of disability, frailty, and comorbidity: implications for improved targeting and care. J Gerontol A Biol Sci Med Sci. 2004;59:255–63. [PubMed: 15031310]).
11. Bandeen-Roche K, Xue Q-L, Ferrucci L, et al. Phenotype of frailty: characterization in the women's health and aging studies. J Gerontol. 2006;61A(3):262–6.
12. Aprahamian I, De Castro N, Izbicki R. Screening for frailty scale: a comparison with the phenotype criteria. JAMDA. 2017;18(7):592–6.

Chapter 2
Frailty Assessment

Angela Benjumea

Frailty is a condition that places older persons at risk of poor outcomes when exposed to stressful events. Frailty is present in approximately 5% of the population aged 60 and older. Numerous studies have suggested that frailty is a predictor of functional deterioration and mortality. Models of frailty have been developed using three different domains: functional, deficit accumulation, and biological [1]. Frailty represents a potential public health problem due to the multiple clinical and social consequences and its dynamic nature. Identifying frail older adults or those at risk of frailty should be one of the foundations of geriatric care, since it is a complex and important issue associated with aging, with implications for both the patients and the health services. Adequate recognition of frailty may reduce risks from possibly detrimental interventions, being currently unacceptable to consider patients' risk only on their chronological age. The dynamic nature of frailty highlights a potential for preventive and restorative interventions, so that when detected early, it is possible to preserve the functional and cognitive reserves, to maintain the capacity for self-care and to prevent disabilities, falls, functional decline, institutionalization, hospitalization, and death [2]. There are a growing number of instruments that aim to evaluate frailty.

In 2001, Fried and colleagues proposed their landmark frailty phenotype measurement, (the CHS index), which assessed frailty by measuring five of its physical components. Following this, and also in 2001, Rockwood and Mitnitski released their accumulated deficits model of frailty, which considered not only the physical components of frailty, but also the psychosocial aspects of frailty. Both of these frailty models are highly regarded and used today. Nowadays, a plethora of frailty measuring tools are in existence. Identifying which frailty measuring tool is most suitable for clinical and/or research application is currently a topic of heated debate. Moreover, multiple reviews have highlighted the need for a standard measurement

A. Benjumea (✉)
Faculty of Health Sciences, Caldas University, Caldas, Colombia
e-mail: angela.benjumea@ucaldas.edu.co

© Springer Nature Switzerland AG 2021

C. G. Musso et al. (eds.), *Frailty and Kidney Disease*,
https://doi.org/10.1007/978-3-030-53529-2_2

of frailty in research and/or clinical practice. A standard measurement would allow for consistent recognition of frailty worldwide [3]. Dent and colleagues, summarized the main strengths and limitations of existing frailty measuring tools, and examined how well these measurements operationalized frailty according to Clegg's guidelines for frailty classification, their accuracy in identifying frailty, their basis on biological causative theory, and their ability to reliably predict patients' outcomes and their response to potential therapies. Four hundred twenty-two studies were identified. From these studies, 29 different frailty measurements were identified. Overall, frailty measurements were used for frailty classification and prognosis across a broad range of medical patients, including geriatric, oncology, surgical, orthopedic, cardiovascular, and renal patients. This review showed that there are multiple measuring tools used to identify frailty in older people. There was a wide range in the applicability of these frailty measuring tools: from short, fast and crude frailty screening instruments to the sophisticated, time-consuming measurements. Many frailty measuring tools had not been robustly validated in the literature, and their prognostic ability was rarely determined. Moreover, many frailty measuring tools were modified somewhat from their original, validated version, which in turn, can have a striking impact on frailty classification. The majority of these medical studies used frailty measurement as a prognostic tool, applying Fried's frailty phenotype and the frailty index (FI) [3]. Frailty is considered as an at-risk state caused by the age-associated accumulation of deficits. A method has been proposed for how a frailty index can be derived from existing health databases by proposing criteria for deficits and procedures for counting deficits. The current concept is that the number of deficits is important: the more deficits individuals accumulate, the more they are at risk of an adverse health outcome, which means that with more deficits, they are at more risk and, then they are more frail. In this sense, deficit accumulation is indistinguishable from the loss of physiologic reserve, being a convenient way for geriatricians to record and count deficits to use the information gathered as part of a routine comprehensive geriatric assessment (CGA). Then, the frailty index was constructed as an index based on a comprehensive geriatric assessment (FI-CGA). The total number of items that can be used in a frailty index is considered to be 80, assuming that the maximum number of diagnoses is 15 and the maximum number of medications is 20. In this sense, for any individual, a frailty index score based on CGA is calculated as the number of deficits that he/she has, divided by the total number of deficits that were considered (e.g.: 80) For instance, a woman with diabetes mellitus, peptic ulcer disease, osteoarthritis, hypothyroidism, and osteoporosis, (5 deficits), who takes 7 medications (1 deficit); needs help with banking, shopping, and transportation (3 deficits); complains of anxiety; rates her health as only fair; and seems poorly motivated to change her health status (2 deficits) would have 11 deficits. Therefore, her frailty index score would be the 11 deficits she has, divided by the 80 deficits that were considered, that is, an FI-CGA score of 11/80 = 0.14. Since the patient's deficit accumulation is highly correlated with the risk of death, it is possible to consider this deficit accumulation as an estimated patient's biological age. Consider two people, A and B, who have both 78 years of age, at this age the mean value of the frailty index is 0.16. However, person A has a frailty index value of 0.26, which is in fact the frailty index corresponding to a 93 years old person. Thus, person A has a life expectancy corresponding to a 93 years old individual, which means that he/she has a chronological age of 78 years, but a biological age of 93 years. Conversely, person B has a frailty index value of 0.1, which is a lower value than the expected one, being this frailty index corresponding to a 63 year old individual. Thus, in essence, person B has a life expectancy corresponding to a 63 years old individual, which means that he/she has a chronological age of 78 years, and a biological age of 63 years. Therefore, it is proposed this approach to measure patients' biological age, since research studies have confirmed the high correlation between mortality and deficit accumulation [4].

Many frailty instruments are useful for identifying high risk individuals for adverse outcomes, but less for developing clinical interventions to prevent or treat frailty. Additionally, agreement between these instruments has been shown to vary greatly. Maintaining validity in terms of ensuring that instruments are measuring their intended frailty-related constructs is another important consideration. Because short and simple instruments for detecting frailty are most feasible in clinical practice, several quick screening tools have been developed and validated for this purpose: [5].

1. *Clinical Frailty Scale (CFS)*: The Clinical Frailty Scale (CFS) is a well validated frailty measuring tool created by Dalhousie University in Canada. It is scored on a scale from 1 (very fit) to 9 (terminally ill), and is based on clinical judgment. Each point on its scale corresponds with a written description of frailty, complemented by a visual chart to assist with the classification of frailty. A score ≥5 is considered to be frail. The CFS can be extracted from data from medical charts, and therefore can also be derived from CGAs. The CFS has been validated as an adverse outcome predictor in hospitalized older people [6–8].
2. *Edmonton Frailty Scale (EFS)*: The Edmonton Frailty Scale (EFS) is a validated and reliable measuring tool for frailty identification in the hospital setting. The EFS is scored out of 17, and contains nine components: cognition, general health status, self-reported health, functional independence, social support, polypharmacy, mood, continence, and functional performance. Component scores are summed, and the following cut-off score is used to classify frailty severity: not frail (0–5), apparently vulnerable [6, 7], mildly frail [8, 9], moderately frail [10, 11], and severely frailty [12–17]. With only nine components, the EFS is much simpler to extract from CGAs than the FI-CGA. The EFS is increasingly being used to identify frailty in specific clinical populations, and an adapted version, the Reported EFS has been developed for acute care [9–12].
3. *Fatigue, Resistance, Ambulation, Illness, Loss of Weight (FRAIL) Index*: Recently proposed by the International Association of Nutrition and Ageing (IANA), FRAIL is comprised of five components: Fatigue (self-report), Resistance, Ambulation (slow walking speed), Illness, and Loss of weight (5% or more in the past year). When three or more of these components are present, an older

person is classified as frail. FRAIL is judged to be clinically advantageous due to its simple nature and ability to be obtained from data already included in a patient CGA. It has been found to be predictive of mortality in specific populations. Further validation studies of FRAIL are needed for both hospitalized and community dwelling older people [1, 13, 14].

4. *Study of Osteoporotic Fractures (SOF) Index*: The Study of Osteoporotic Fractures (SOF) frailty index, like the CHS index, considers frailty to be phenotypic in nature, with an underlying biological causative theory. The SOF is easy to apply, with frailty classified as the presence of ≥2 components out of list of three: weight loss (intentional/unintentional, 5% in the last year), exhaustion (an answer of 'no' to the question 'do you feel full of energy?'), and low mobility (inability to perform a five-times-chair-rise test). The SOF is valid and reliable, and has been found to be an independent predictor of adverse outcomes in community-dwelling older people. It generally compares well to the FI and the CHS regarding adverse outcome prediction. The SOF is suited for both population screening and clinical assessment, although it tends to over-screen frailty in the hospital setting because patients with an acute medical condition often cannot perform a five-times-chair-rise test [15–17].
5. *Mobility performance tests:* Five-chair sit-to-stand (STS): This test measured the time taken to stand from a sitting position five times without using the arms. Patients were asked to stand up and sit down on a straight-backed chair (they sat on a chair that was 46 cm high) as quickly as possible. The time was measured from the initial sitting position to the final fully erect position at the end of the fifth stand up. Timed chair standing is a reliable and valid test that reflects older adults' lower extremity muscle force, balance, and functional mobility [18].

Alternate step: This test involves weight shifting and provides a measure of lateral stability. Patients were asked to step alternately eight times with each leg onto a raised platform (19 cm high). The time taken to alternately place each foot on a 19 cm high step eight times was measured. Alternate step test has been found to be a valid, reliable, and feasible clinical test for measuring mobility [18].

TUG: This test measured the time to rise from a 46-cm high chair, walk forward by 3 meters as quickly as possible, turn by 180°, walk back to the chair, and sit down. This test has been found to be a reliable and valid test for quantifying functional mobility [18].

TRG: This test measured the time to walk back and forth over a 10-foot course as quickly as possible. The feasibility of the rapid gait test in clinical practice has been demonstrated. Timing was started when a participant was ready and tester said "go" and was stopped when the participant's first foot crossed the starting line [18].

UGS: Gait speed test may be the best indicator of frailty among all of Fried's frailty components. Importantly, gait speed also has a close association with adverse health outcomes in older people. Gait speed is applicable clinically, although it does over-screen for frailty, and there are fundamental difficulties in measuring out walking course in a clinical setting [19].

Grip Strength (GS): Low grip strength can also be used as a single measure of frailty, and has been found to be predictive of both functional decline and long stay in hospitalized older patients, and mortality in community dwelling adults. It has also been found to be a good marker of poor mobility [20–23].

In conclusion, there are a lot of frailty measuring tools, although a qualified frailty measurement should be able not only to identify this syndrome, but also to predict patients' outcomes, their response to potential treatments, and have biological bases. Based on these criteria, the two most robust frailty assessment tools, commonly used by clinicians and researchers are Fried's Frailty Phenotype (the CHS index) and Rockwood and Mitnitski's Frailty Index (FI). Frailty measurement should be incorporated into clinical practice as part of routine care for older patients.

References

1. Malmstrom T, Miller D, Morley J. A comparison of four frailty models. J Am Geriatr Soc. 2014;62(4):721–6. https://doi.org/10.1111/jgs.12735.
2. Wilke J, Nascimiento D, Souza S. Instruments for the detection of frailty syndrome in older adults: a systematic review. PLoS One. 2019;14(4):e0216166. https://doi.org/10.1371/journal.pone.0216166.
3. Dent E, Kowal P, Hoogendijk E. Frailty measurement in research and clinical practice: a review. Eur J InternMed. 2016;31:3–10. https://doi.org/10.1016/j.ejim.2016.03.007.
4. Rockwood K, Mitnitski A. Frailty defined by deficit accumulation and geriatric medicine defined by frailty. Clin Geriatr Med. 2011;27:17–26. https://doi.org/10.1016/j.cger.2010.08.008.
5. Waltson J, Buta B, Xue Q. Frailty screening and interventions. Clin Geriatr Med. 2018;34:25–38. https://doi.org/10.1016/j.cger.2017.09.004.
6. Rockwood K, Song X, MacKnight C, et al. A global clinical measure of fitness and frailty in elderly people. CMAJ. 2005;173(5):489–95.
7. Basic D, Shanley C. Frailty in an older inpatient population: using the clinical frailty scale to predict patient outcomes. J Aging Health. 2015;27(4):670–85.
8. Wallis SJ, Wall J, Biram RW, Romero-Ortuno R. Association of the clinical frailty scale with hospital outcomes. QJM. 2015;108(12):943–9.
9. Rolfson DB, Majumdar SR, Tsuyuki RT, Tahir A, Rockwood K. Validity and reliability of the Edmonton frail scale. Age Ageing. 2006;35(5):526–9.
10. Partridge JS, Fuller M, Harari D, Taylor PR, Martin FC, Dhesi JK. Frailty and por functional status are common in arterial vascular surgical patients and affect postoperative outcomes. Int J Surg. 2015;18:57–63.
11. Graham MM, Galbraith PD, O'Neill D, Rolfson DB, Dando C, Norris CM. Frailty and outcome in elderly patients with acute coronary syndrome. Can J Cardiol. 2013;29(12):1610–5.
12. Hilmer SN, Perera V, Mitchell S, Murnion BP, Dent J, Bajorek B, et al. The assessment of frailty in older people in acute care. Australas J Ageing. 2009;28(4):182–8.
13. Morley JE, Malmstrom TK, Miller DK. A simple frailty questionnaire (FRAIL) predicts outcomes in middle aged African Americans. J Nutr Health Aging. 2012;16(7):601–8.
14. Woo J, Leung J, Morley JE. Comparison of frailty indicators based on clinical phenotype and the multiple deficit approach in predicting mortality and physical limitation. J Am Geriatr Soc. 2012;60(8):1478–86.
15. Ensrud KE, Ewing SK, Taylor BC, Fink HA, Stone KL, Cauley JA, et al. Frailty and risk of falls, fracture, and mortality in older women: the study of osteoporotic fractures. J Gerontol A Biol Sci Med Sci. 2007;62(7):744–51.

16. Bilotta C, Nicolini P, Case A, Pina G, Rossi S, Vergani C. Frailty syndrome diagnosed according to the study of osteoporotic fractures (SOF) criteria and adverse health outcomes among community-dwelling older outpatients in Italy. A one-year prospective cohort study. Arch Gerontol Geriatr. 2012;54(2):e23–8.
17. Ensrud KE, Ewing SK, Cawthon PM, Fink HA, Taylor BC, Cauley JA, et al. A comparison of frailty indexes for the prediction of falls, disability, fractures, and mortality in older men. J Am Geriatr Soc. 2009;57(3):492–8.
18. Kim M, Yabushita N, Kim M, et al. Mobility Performance Test for discriminating high risk of frailty in community-dwelling older women. Arch Gerontol Geriatr. 2010;51:192–8.
19. Toots A, Rosendahl E, Lundin-Olsson L, Nordstrom P, Gustafson Y, Littbrand H. Usual gait speed independently predicts mortality in very old people: a population-based study. J Am Med Dir Assoc. 2013;14(7):529, [e521–526.]
20. Garcia-Pena C, Garcia-Fabela LC, Gutierrez-Robledo LM, Garcia-Gonzalez JJ, Arango-Lopera VE, Perez-Zepeda MU. Handgrip strength predicts functional decline at discharge in hospitalized male elderly: a hospital cohort study. PLoS One. 2013;8(7):e69849.
21. Roberts HC, Syddall HE, Cooper C, Aihie Sayer A. Is grip strength associated with length of stay in hospitalised older patients admitted for rehabilitation? Findings from the Southampton grip strength study. Age Ageing. 2012;41(5):641–6.
22. Leong DP, Teo KK, Rangarajan S, Lopez-Jaramillo P, Avezum A Jr, Orlandini A, et al. Prognostic value of grip strength: findings from the prospective urban rural epidemiology (PURE) study. Lancet. 2015;386(9990):266–73.
23. Stevens PJ, Syddall HE, Patel HP, Martin HJ, Cooper C, Aihie Sayer A. Is grip strength a good marker of physical performance among community-dwelling older people? J Nutr Health Aging. 2012;16(9):769–74.

Chapter 3
Falls and Gait Disorders in Older Adults: Causes and Consequences

Manuel Montero-Odasso and Tahir Masud

Introduction

Over the course of the aging process, there is an increased risk for falling and therefore subsequent adverse consequences including soft tissue and bone injury, disability, dependency, premature nursing home admission, and mortality [1]. This trend has been well established for many years and was first described nearly 40 years ago in the context of one of the so-called "geriatric giants" termed *Instability*. Falls and concomitant fall-related injuries in older people are a prevalent and global issue that pose substantial clinical and public health implications [2].

A fall is defined as "an unintentional change in position resulting in coming to rest at a lower level or on the ground" [3]. It is important to note that syncope and loss of consciousness due to seizures or an acute stroke are not included in the fall definition despite the fact that they also often present as an episode of instability and a change of position to a lower level [4, 5]. From an etiological standpoint, falls generally have multiple and diverse causes and frequently result from the accumulated effect of impairments in multiple systems, illustrating their complexity.

M. Montero-Odasso (✉)
Departments of Medicine, and Epidemiology and Biostatistics, The University of Western Ontario, London, ON, Canada

Division of Geriatric Medicine, Parkwood Institute, The University of Western Ontario, London, ON, Canada

Lawson Health Research Institute, London, ON, Canada

Gait and Brain Lab, Parkwood Institute, London, ON, Canada
e-mail: mmontero@uwo.ca

T. Masud
Nottingham University Hospitals NHS Trust, Nottingham, UK
e-mail: tahir.masud@nuh.nhs.uk

© Springer Nature Switzerland AG 2021

C. G. Musso et al. (eds.), *Frailty and Kidney Disease*,
https://doi.org/10.1007/978-3-030-53529-2_3

Falls as a "Geriatric Giant"

For centuries, falling has been described as a natural accident that occurs commonly as a geriatric syndrome in older adults. In its initial inception, falls management was focused only on the mechanical consequences of the fall, namely the physical injury resulting from the fall. The geriatric giants known as *"Instability"* and *"Immobility"* include falls and fractures as critical components [6], and both are important in the vicious cycle of falls and fractures in older adults. As depicted in Fig. 3.1, once the individual feels immobilized as a result of previous falls, there is development of further neuromuscular impairment, which in turn, often leads to muscle weakness, sarcopenia, and deconditioning that further increases the risk of future falls and fractures. It is therefore apparent that falls are both a cause and a consequence of neuromuscular and physical impairment. This trend was first described in observational studies conducted in the early1980s, illustrating the epidemiology, consequences, and underlying factors responsible for the occurrence of recurrent falls, and is sometimes referred to as the *falls syndrome* [2, 3, 5, 7–10]. Following this initial description, clinical trials were conducted in the late 1980s demonstrating that multifactorial and multidisciplinary interventions that target a series of lifestyle factors may be best suited in preventing falls and their concomitant consequences [2, 11–15].

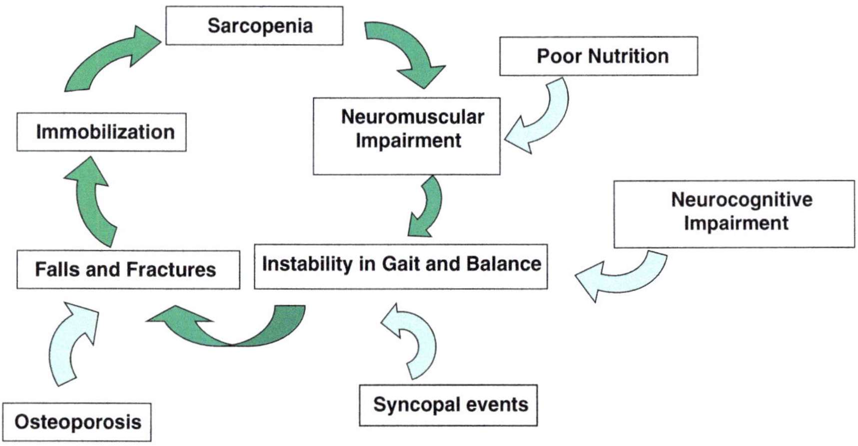

Fig. 3.1 Vicious cycle in falls with principal contributors. Modified from Montero-Odasso [84]. Green arrows represent the cycle. Light blue arrows represent the contributors

Table 3.1 Incidence rate of falls by population type

Population description	Annual incidence rate of future falls
Community dwelling older adults aged 65 years or older [14]	30%
Older adults hospitalized as patients [16–18]	40%
Community dwelling older adults aged 80 years or older [14]	40–50%
Older adults living in long-term care facilities [16–18]	45–50%
Individuals with a history of falls in the previous year [16–18]	60%

Note. Numbers accompanying population description are the references

It is now well established that the risk of falling is strongly linked with age, as after the sixth decade of life (age 60 or older), the incidence of falls rises steadily with further aging and reaches its highest incidence rate among persons aged 80 years or older. Comorbidities commonly associated with the natural aging process include osteoporosis, visual impairment, and the loss of adaptive and defensive mechanisms related to falls prevention. These comorbidities place older adults at greater risk of sustaining a serious injury, even after the occurrence of a minor fall. This inability to prevent fall accidents is of critical importance, as accidents are ranked in the top five leading causes of death in high income countries and falls are considered the single leading cause of accidental death in older adults [16] (see Table 3.1).

But despite the general trends delineated above, there are important differences in the prevalence and incidence of falls depending on the population and setting under observation. Table 3.1 describes the incidence rates of falls in various populations.

Evidently, factors such as hospitalization and age contribute to the increase in future falls risk. But importantly, history of falls in the past year poses a considerable risk of future falls which is concerning, as falls constitute the largest single cause of injury related mortality in older adults. Moreover, falls independently determine the risk of functional decline, and account for, approximately, 40% of all nursing home admissions and substantial societal costs [17].

Consequences of Falling

There is a plethora of serious medical, psychological, and social consequences resulting from the occurrence of falls, many of which are underreported or underestimated in the literature (see Table 3.2).

As depicted in Table 3.2, the consequences of falls are debilitating, regardless of the cause, and can potentially result in death.

Table 3.2 Frequent consequences of the fall syndrome in older people

Cause	Consequence
Medical/Physical	Head trauma
	Soft-tissue hematoma
	Fracture
	Joint dislocation
	Chronic pain
	Death
Psychological	Fear of falling
	Anxiety
	Loss of confidence
	Depression
Social	Dependency
	Isolation
	Placement in long-term care
Functional	Immobility
	Deconditioning
	Disability and dependence

Morbidity and Mortality

Falls are the leading cause of death from trauma and injury in men and women aged 65 years and older. Following the occurrence of a fall, a cascade of additional psychological and medical consequences follows. Not surprisingly, 20% of those who have had a previous fall will develop a "fear of falling," 15% will sustain an injury that leads to visits to an emergency department, 10% will sustain a severe injury but not a fracture (e.g., head injury, brain hematomas, or chest trauma), 5% will sustain a fracture, and 1% a hip fracture [17, 18]. For higher risk individuals, such as women 75 years of age and older [19] and cognitively impaired older adults [20], these percentages are more than doubled.

In addition to factors outlined such as hospitalization, increased age, and cognitive impairment, the *way* an individual falls is also related to the type of injury that they will sustain. For example, falling forward usually results in a wrist or hand fracture, and wrist fractures are also more prevalent in older adults between the ages of 65–75. Falling on one's side is more likely to result in hip fractures, and hip fractures are most prevalent in individuals over the age of 75. Falling backwards tends to have the lowest rate of resulting fractures. Notably, not only the *way* one falls, but also an individual's age predicts whether or not they sustain no injury, a wrist fracture, or a hip fracture, with the latter being more common in older age. Several hypotheses have been postulated in an attempt to explain this age-related shift from wrist to hip fractures. For instance, it has been suggested that individuals over 75 years of age have slower defensive reflexes than their younger counterparts, and are thus at greater risk for falling in ways that result in more pronounced injuries such as pelvis and hip fractures [21].

Psychological and Social Consequences

Although the physical consequences of falls are of critical importance, no less important are the psychological and social consequences of falls. As previously alluded, "fear of falling" is common in individuals who have experienced a single fall and is highly common in individuals who have had recurrent falls [17, 22–24]. This anxiety and fear of falling can significantly impact their quality of life.

Fear of falling and anxiety can lead to isolation, as individuals may be reluctant to engage in various activity types. This isolation from activities and daily experience of fear and anxiety can further lead to depression and poor life satisfaction. Surprisingly, fear of falling has been shown to be a predictor of future falls, indicating that despite the efforts made to avoid falls by individuals with a fear of falling—their anxiety about falling may actually cause rather than prevent future falls. It appears that fear of experiencing another fall (known as "post fall anxiety") may trigger a downward spiral, negatively influencing an individual's social and psychological wellbeing. This impact on their psychological wellbeing thereby reduces their participation in social activities and isolates them which may directly contribute to their feelings of loneliness and hopelessness, and potentially lead to a diagnosis of depression.

Risk Factors for Falls

While it may be possible to determine the direct trigger for a given fall, the actual underlying causes of falls in older persons are varied and complex. Multiple risk factors for falls have been identified including those discussed thus far in this chapter such as age-related decline of bodily functions including sensory impairment and neuromuscular weakness. In addition to these, comorbidities such as cardiovascular disease, polypharmacy, and environmental hazards have been identified as common risk factors for falls [8, 25, 26]. Of course, environmental hazards pose a fundamentally different risk to individuals than do internal comorbidities and medical conditions. For example, an individual who is cognitively intact, medically healthy, and has excellent sensory functioning may have a high risk of falls simply due to a high prevalence of environmental hazards that may cause her/him to trip, slip, and fall. Thus, the most accepted classification of falls pertains to whether the risk factors for the fall are related to an extrinsic hazard or an intrinsic disorder [16, 27]. *Extrinsic falls* are typically related to environmental hazards causing individuals to slip, trip, or sustain an externally induced displacement, whereas *intrinsic falls* include mobility or balance disorders, muscle weakness, orthopedic problems, sensory impairment, or a neurally-mediated cardiovascular disorder such as postural hypotension or post-prandial hypotension [27]. However, for the majority (80%) of fallers, this classification has limited clinical applicability, as their falls are caused by a combination of intrinsic and extrinsic factors [28].

In order to reduce the occurrence of falls, it is important to modify the underlying risk factors. While modifying one risk factor may reduce the incidence of falls, the risk reduction is likely to be greatest when multiple risk factors are modified [15]. Therefore, from a clinical point of view, it is most advantageous and efficient to select interventions that target several risk factors simultaneously.

In this chapter, risk factors are aggregated into four domains as follows, which each relate to the potential interventions as listed in Table 3.5: (1) neuromuscular, (2) medical, (3) cardiovascular, and (4) environmental.

The risk factors for a fall under a given domain may include both medical diagnoses as well as their concomitant symptoms. For example, neuromuscular falls may be caused by Parkinsonism, a neurological diagnosis, as well as lower extremity weakness, a symptom of that diagnosis. It is noteworthy that under medical problems, medications are included, as they are an important cause of falls. There is strong evidence that in addition to the total number of medications taken, both the type and class of medications are important in producing side effects that may cause falls. For example, psychotropics, sedatives, and vasodilators are recognized as contributing to the risk of falling in older adults [22, 29–31]. In two seminal reviews of the literature, Leipzig et al. conducted meta-analyses of studies on falls completed by 1999 [30, 31] identifying by drug classes their attributable risk and odds ratios (OR) for falls each drug group. The use of sedatives, hypnotics, antidepressants, and benzodiazepines increased risk of falls by approximately 1.5 times (with an OR ranging from 1.32 to 1.8). Further details pertaining to each medication type are provided below.

Antianxiety/Hypnotics Medications

Regardless of their duration of action, benzodiazepines have consistently been shown to have a strong dose-response relationship with increased risk of falls, as benzodiazepine users had an adjusted OR = 1.48 (95% CI 1.23, 1.77) for falls.

Antipsychotic Medications

Although their use and prescription is still controversial, antipsychotic medications are widely used to manage some behavioral and psychiatric symptoms in older patients. Atypical antipsychotics are preferred because they have fewer extrapyramidal side effects relative to other antipsychotic medications, but even these confer a risk of future falls. Antipsychotics are associated with a significantly greater risk of falling, with adjusted ORs ranging from 1.30 to 1.74. What this suggests is that individuals who take antipsychotic medications are nearly two times more likely to fall than those who do not take such medications.

Antidepressant Medications

There are generally two classes of medications prescribed for individuals suffering from depression—selective serotonin reuptake inhibitors (SSRIs) and tricyclic antidepressants (TCAs). Recent studies have focused on comparing the falls risk associated with the use of each type. The evidence suggests the risk of falls or hip fractures does not differ between those who use of SSRIs in preference to TCAs, being high for both classes [32, 33].

Antipsychotics and Opioids

In studies of older community dwelling adults, the use of combined central nervous system medications including benzodiazepines, opioid receptor agonists, antipsychotics, and antidepressants appears to increase both the risk of first falls and recurrent falls (adjusted OR = 2.89) [34]. More recent data further support these findings, as a systematic review and meta-analysis in 2018 also found that antipsychotics, antidepressants, and benzodiazepines are consistently associated with an increased risk of falls [35]. What these data suggest is that combining medications that act on the central nervous system confers a significantly higher risk of recurrent falls than the individual medication.

Antihypertensive and Other Cardiovascular Medications

Antihypertensives and cardiovascular medications also appear to increase the risk of falls. The Leipzig et al. [30, 31] meta-analysis identified digoxin, type 1a antiarrhythmics and diuretics as being associated with an increased falls risk. These results are further bolstered by similar findings from a prospective study with 979 rural-dwelling older adults aged 70 years or over in Finland [36]. This study found that injurious falls had a significantly high occurrence in men taking digoxin (OR = 2.2) and any user of calcium channel blockers (OR = 2.4).

Pathophysiology of Falls

A Model for the Understanding of the Basics of Postural Control

There is a certain degree of natural instability due to the anatomical properties of the human upright position. Specifically, when we stand, our feet provide us with a narrow base of support and our mid-section gives us a high center of gravity. Together, these physical properties of human anatomy contribute to a large degree of instability. While standing or walking, the human body needs to maintain a delicate equilibrium via a harmonious modulation of trunk/ankle flexibility. Motor impairments increase the risk of falling by challenging this equilibrium modulation. Physiological perturbations such as body sway during standing or walking or after an extrinsic destabilizing factor such as during tripping also challenge this delicate equilibrium. When a perturbation with a potential to cause a fall occurs, a rapid succession of strategies aimed at preserving body stability follow, the first of which is the "ankle strategy". The ankle strategy is a motor plan characterized by the release of trunk muscles and stiffening of the ankle joint [37–40]. This ankle strategy may not be sufficient during more severe perturbations, and thus a second motor plan, the "stepping strategy" is activated. Here the ankle joint is released, and the individual performs one or more steps to enlarge their base of support. If both, the ankle and stepping motor strategies fail to preserve stability, the upper limbs come into play, performing rescue strategies such reaching out for support or protective reactions including limiting the traumatic consequence of falling when it cannot be avoided. As illustrated by this sequential model, there is a strong pathophysiological link between trunk inflexibility and instability. This model also helps illustrate the clear mechanistic link between gait disorders and falling (i.e., "stepping strategy"). Finally, this model explains the need for an adequate flow of information through visual, vestibular, and somatosensory afferent pathways as well as the need for attentive and executive resources to adapt to the environmental perturbation by rapidly switching from one strategy to the other. Figure 3.2 schematizes these strategies and the role of executive function in controlling and modulating the three classic rescue strategies.

The motor determinants of a frequent faller are characterized by a disorder of either the base of support or the center of body mass [37]. Parkinson's disease (PD) is an example of a common base of support disorder, as patients with PD manifest disorders of both the base of support and the center of body mass. Moreover, individuals with advanced PD fall frequently. PD is generally regarded as a disorder of the brain's dopaminergic system; however, additional processes not strictly confined to the dopaminergic systems may also play a role in the pathogenesis of motor axial impairment. Mild Parkinsonian signs have also been recognized in older adults without PD. These patients present features that are recognized as risk factors for falling, including gait and postural instability and impaired executive cognitive function. The emergence of mild Parkinsonian signs related to vascular lesions mainly involve the frontal regions of the brain [41], supporting the hypothesis that

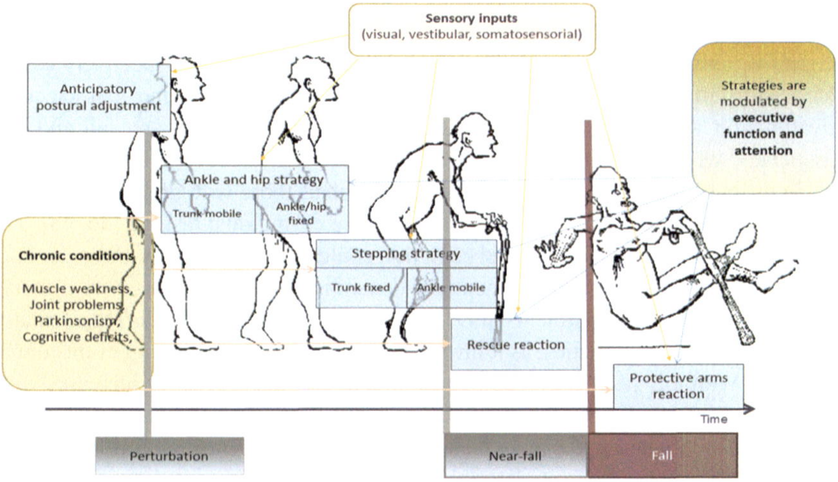

Fig. 3.2 Schematization of rapid succession of strategies aimed at preserving body stability after a single perturbation. Note the role of cognitive processes, attention and executive functions, modulating the three classic rescue strategies. (Reproduced with permission from Montero-Odasso and Speechley [85]

brain cortical control of gait shares the same neural networks of important frontal lobe functions including executive functioning [41].

Cognitive Aspects of Falls Risk: The Role of the Gait and Cognition Interaction in Falls

The view that walking is an entirely automatic motor task is now being challenged as being over simplistic [42]. In the real world, walking requires a myriad of attentional resources including constant avoidance of various environmental hazards and consistent recovering from postural perturbations to avoid stumbles or falls. Unsurprisingly then, attentional deficits and problems with executive functioning are independently associated with an increased risk of postural instability, impairment in activities of daily living, and future falls [43].

There is now a growing body of research on dual-tasking gait (DTG), which is the simultaneous performance of a secondary task while walking. This research has been largely driven by the observation that the failure to maintain a conversation while walking (“stop walking when talking”) is a strong predictor of future falls [44]. With impairments in attentional and cognitive abilities, dual-task abilities worsen as well. Even while standing, postural sway increases when a cognitive task is being performed concurrently. This suggests that the constant dynamic control of postural adjustments during standing inherently requires a certain level of cognitive and attentional resources. Similarly, locomotion also requires a certain degree of attentional resources. In otherwise healthy older adults who present with "normal" cognitive abilities, executive functioning abilities have been prospectively associated with falls [45]. A systematic review and meta-analysis found that executive dysfunction was associated with a 1.44 times increased risk of any fall and falls associated with serious injury [20].

In patients with overt neurological disease such as those with previous incidences of stroke, PD, or dementia, gait deteriorates more during dual tasking [46–48]. This strong association between gait and cognition could explain why falls are so common in patients with cognitive impairment and dementia and why patients with dementia are so vulnerable to impairments in DTG performance. Dual tasking is representative of regular daily life activities, as it involves many attention-demanding events during walking. With this perspective, it is unsurprising that fall frequency increases while performing a secondary attention-demanding task, as cognitive resources are utilized for the secondary task and cannot be as readily available to prevent falls.

Finally, further evidence bolstering the notion that attention and cognition play a pivotal role in postural control comes from the fact that medications that impair cognitive abilities also increase the risk of falls. In contrast to medications that impair cognitive abilities, cognitive enhancers (including the cholinesterase inhibitor donepezil, used for the treatment of dementia) *reduce* falls significantly. Although it may appear as though the medications themselves reduced falls, this is unlikely, as patients with PD who do *not* have cognitive impairment often present with near-falls rather than actual falls, suggesting that medications used to treat dementia may not themselves improve stability, but rather cognitive resources improve stability. Taken together, these findings imply that medications that enhance cognitive resources subsequently reduce falls. Similarly, cognitive enhancers have improved gait and mobility in people with Alzheimer's disease [49, 50].

Risk Identification

Falls Classification and the Role of Gait Assessments

Falls can be classified in a number of diverse ways including by their number (single fall vs. multiple falls); whether or not an injury was sustained (injurious falls vs. non-injurious falls); and what risk factors may have been involved (intrinsic vs. extrinsic factors). The traditional classification based on the presence of intrinsic and extrinsic factors is widely used, validated, and accepted worldwide [27]. However, when used in isolation, its utility is limited, as it is difficult to attribute a fall to an extrinsic factor alone, given that the majority of environmentally related falls result from a complex interaction between extrinsic and intrinsic risk factors. The intrinsic-extrinsic categorization was originally developed in order to separate and delineate multiple contributions to a given fall. However, it is noteworthy that older people who experience an extrinsic fall often have an underlying intrinsic condition that decreases their ability to compensate for the hazardous situation which originally may have caused the initiation of the fall. One of the themes of this chapter is that falls are multifaceted in their cause and often result from a complex interaction between factors that challenge both the individual's postural control and their ability to maintain an upright position.

Gait and balance difficulties are commonly associated with the aging process that confers profound negative impacts on a person's health and quality of life [22, 51–53]. There are a number of individual disorders of aging that affect mobility and gait in older persons including loss of muscle mass and strength (e.g., sarcopenia), decreases in visual acuity, impairment in proprioception, and impairments in nerve conduction with a resultant loss of defense reflexes. In addition to these age-related physiological impairments, many chronic diseases and conditions such as arthritis, neurological problems, and cardiac and respiratory conditions often have marked effects on gait and balance [54, 55]. Not only physiological diseases and conditions themselves, but symptoms such as chronic pain, dizziness and reduced joint mobility may also contribute to an increased risk of falling [51].

In order to successfully walk (i.e., gait performance), a multitude of systems must work in coordination and harmony with one other [51, 56]. Because impairments in different domains can alter this delicate system, it has been hypothesized that chronic conditions that increase fall risk such as visual or hearing problems, muscular weakness, osteoarthritis, or peripheral neuropathy could be identified through gait performance assessment [56]. Gait disorders are among the highest predictive risk factor for falls in older adults [5, 51, 56, 57].

In clinical practice, assessment of gait is recommended to identify significant risk factors that generate the individual's increased fall risk. In addition to identifying modifiable fall risk factors on which to build a plan to prevent future falls, it can help to diagnose rarer single treatable conditions such as myelopathy and normal pressure hydrocephalus which may be contributing to an individual's fall risk.

One simple method of doing this is to routinely perform gait assessment as a regular clinical observation procedure. Formal testing in a gait laboratory with expensive equipment is not necessary, as gait assessments can be done in typical clinical and medical settings quite readily. However, the kind of high-tech analysis in gait laboratories might be useful in select cases such as when developing a specific rehabilitation strategy, measuring changes in gait quantitative markers, and for specific research purposes. A focused and careful observation of gait performance can detect subtle abnormalities and underlying impairments, which can thereby identify the pathologic process involved. Table 3.3 describes some of the common

Table 3.3 Common symptoms of falls, abnormal mobility, and gait in older adults in relation to a performance-based evaluation

Symptom	Potential cause
Difficulty rising from a chair	Lower limb weakness
	Osteoarthritis
Instability on first standing	Postural hypotension
	Muscle weakness
Instability with eyes closed	Proprioception deficits
Decreased step height/length	Parkinsonism
	Frontal lobe disease
	Fear of falling

symptoms associated with falls and gait problems in older adults as well as their relationship to performance-based gait evaluation.

As depicted in Table 3.3, there is not a simple 1:1 relationship between symptoms and potential causes, as often a gait-related symptom has a multitude of potential causes—adding to the complexity of understanding the physiology of gait-related disorders.

Table 3.4 shows that gait impairments can be grouped into three major hierarchical categories as a function of the sensorimotor level involved.

Nutt and Alexander (1993) proposed this classification of gait disorders in older people based on sensorimotor levels [51, 58]. As illustrated in Table 3.4, lower level sensorimotor impairment can be attributed to joint and/or muscular problems and/or peripheral nerve disease; lower extremity motor problems such as chronic pain, joint and foot deformities, or focal muscle weakness are prevalent in seniors and can lead to compensatory changes in gait. Evidence shows that up to 50% of ambulatory older patients seeking a consultation for gait impairment have joint or muscle problems in the lower limbs [59]. Further bolstering this finding was a systematic review of the literature finding that lower limb muscle weakness is significantly associated with falls and subsequent disability in older adults [60]. At a middle sensorimotor level, impaired ability to modulate sensory and motor control of gait occurs without affecting the ignition of walking; typical examples of this include gait disturbances due to PD or due to muscle spasticity associated with hemiplegia. At a high sensorimotor level, gait characteristic become less important, with cognitive impairment, poor attention, and fear of falling playing a more important role as risk factors for falls. This category includes "frontal gait" problems (sometimes referred to as "apraxic gait"), "ignition gait" disturbances, and the "cautious gait" due to fear of falling. Finally, because older adults may have deficits at more than one level, combinations of these levels are frequently observed. Among older adults who present with a gait disturbance, the cause may be easily identifiable, such as PD or a previous stroke with hemiparesis or with a neuropathic foot drop. However, for many older adults with impaired gait, identification of the underlying cause can be challenging. Even in specialized neurology clinics, the underlying cause remained "unknown" in up to 20% of patients attending for gait problems. This was the case even after diagnostic tools such as neuroimaging were used to try to identify the cause [53]. In addition to helping identify causes of falls, an additional value of gait assessments is to help rule out cardiovascular contributors to falls. It has been postulated that falls occurring from neurally-mediated cardiovascular causes may be expressed by a different mechanism, such that they do not necessarily pose any chronic effects on gait performance [57, 61]. Although the exact mechanism by which a neurally-mediated cardiovascular problem causes a fall remains unclear, there is growing clinical evidence for its association with unexplained falls [62]. It is therefore possible to observe older adults who present with recurrent falls but do not have gait problems in which case the consideration of cardiovascular causes should be prompted [63], and cardiac investigations such as tilt testing, echocardiography, and arrhythmia identification event recorders may be required.

Table 3.4 Classifying common causes of gait disorders in older people according to hierarchic level categories

Level	Deficit/condition	Gait characteristic
Low	Peripheral sensory ataxia: posterior column, peripheral nerves, vestibular and visual ataxia	Unsteady, uncoordinated (especially without visual input)
	Peripheral motor deficit due to hip problems	Avoids weight bearing on affected side
	Arthritis (antalgic gait, joint deformity)	Painful knee flexed
		Painful spine produces short slow steps and decreased lumbar lordosis, kyphosis, and ankylosing spondylosis produce stooped posture
	Peripheral motor deficit due to myopathy and neuropathic conditions (weakness)	Proximal motor neuropathy produces waddling and foot slap Distal motor neuropathy produces distal weakness (foot drop)
Middle	Spasticity from hemiplegia, hemiparesis	Leg swings outward and in a semi-circle from hip (circumduction)
	Spasticity from paraplegia, paresis	Circumduction of both legs; steps are short, shuffling, and scraping
	Parkinsonism	Small shuffling steps, hesitation, acceleration (festination), falling forward (propulsion)
	Cerebral ataxia	Wide-based gait with increased trunk sway, irregular stepping
High	Cautious gait	Fear of falling with appropriate postural responses, normal to widened gait base, shortened stride, slower turning "in block". Performance improve with assistance or evaluator walking on the side
	Apraxic gait	Slow gait with short steps due to loss of ability to properly use lower limbs for walking and other, particularly bilateral or abstract motor leg tasks. No apparent strength, cerebellar, proprioception, or vestibular loss
	Frontal-related gait	Frontal gait disorder: short steps length with shuffling gait, like Parkinsonian, but with a wider base, upright posture, and arm swing presence. Gait Ignition failure: difficulty starting these patters has been associated with high white matter disease burden and normal pressure hydrocephalus

Source: Adapted with permission from Nutt et al. [58] and Alexander [51]

Dual-Task Gait Assessments

As alluded to previously in this chapter, dual-task gait assessment has been proposed and used as an instrument to detect the role of cognitive deficits in gross motor performance, gait stability and navigation, and in fall risk assessment. The unique feature of using dual-task gait assessments is that these tests can isolate the

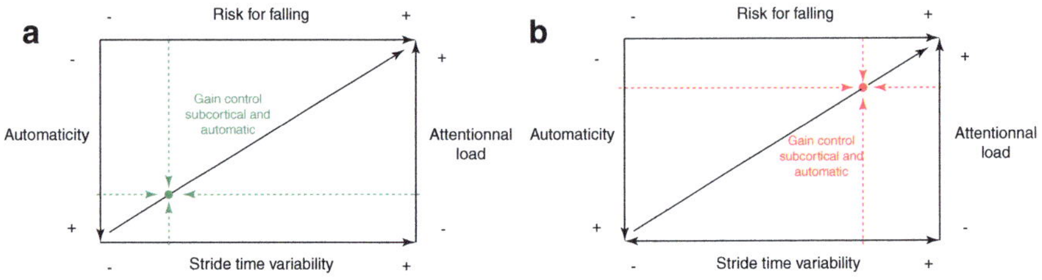

Fig. 3.3 The interplay between gait performance, gait variability, attentional load, and risk of falls. *Note:* Green point in the figure (**a**) represents a more automatic gait that requires less central level of attention and is characterized by low gait variability. Red point in figure (**b**) represents a more instable gait that may occur when control relies more on a high level of attention and executive function, and is characterized by high gait variability

roles of attention and executive functioning deficits in older adults who present with gait control deficits [47, 48, 64]. There is now an emerging body of evidence suggesting that dual-task gait assessments can help identify risk of falls in an individual without previous falls [64].

During the dual-task assessment, individuals are asked to perform an attention-demanding task while walking [65]. The underlying rationale for the use of dual-task gait assessments is that two simultaneously performed tasks interfere and compete for neuro-cortical resources [43]. Figure 3.3 describes how during cases in which attentional demands increase, walking relies more heavily on neural networks that exert higher cortical control. What is considered a "safe gait" occurs when there is more automatic control such that the individual needs to exert a low level of attention and their walk is characterized by low gait variability. Low gait variability simply refers to walking in a manner that is consistent between each stride. When attentional demands increase or when attentional reserves decrease, gait control becomes less automatic, requiring a higher level of attention to be recruited and the individual's walk is then characterized by high gait variability. Given the simultaneous cognitive and motor demands of dual-task gait performance, these assessments can act as a brain stress test which detects impeding mobility problems and can identify the risk of falling. Individuals may alter their gait during dual-tasking (such as by slowing down)—a phenomenon termed "dual-task cost," as it confers an increased cost with involvement of additional cortical and attentional resources while walking. The literature on dual-task cost's ability to serve as a marker of future falls is mixed. This is partly due to the heterogeneity of studies, small sample sizes within individual studies, limited prospective fall ascertainment, and the lack of standardization in dual-task procedures [66, 67]. Although clinically meaningful, cut-off values of dual-task costs for predicting falls are still controversial. Despite this, a growing body of evidence supports the potential clinical utility of dual-task cost measures as a method for falls prediction. The advantages of using dual task gait assessments to predict falls are numerous, as these tests do not require costly equipment, they are not invasive or painful for patients, and they can easily be implemented in practice to provide a valid and sensitive means of assessing motor-cognitive interactions and fall risk. Recent studies indicate that a dual-task cost higher than 20% may suggest that individuals are at higher risk of falls—particularly when they sustain a gait speed of 95 cm/s or faster. These findings highlight the sensitivity and predictive ability of this test in older adults who have a relatively normal gait velocity [66]. Despite these promising findings, Menant and colleagues (2014) conducted a systemic review and meta-analysis and were not able to find the additional value of dual-task gait as a predictor falls over single gait speed [68]. In contrast, a systematic review conducted by Muir-Hunter and colleagues found that in the few studies where both single gait and dual-task gait were assessed, dual-task gait showed added value in predicting future falls [69]. Taken together, it may be advantageous to conduct both single gait and dual-task gait assessments in older individuals to predict future falls risk—as neither assessment is costly nor poses any risks to the individual completing the assessment.

Falls Risk Assessment

Due to the high prevalence of falls in older people and the resulting serious consequences, screening strategies to identify those at high risk of falls have been advocated. A systematic approach has been proposed and recommended as the ideal falls risk assessment using the American Geriatrics Society, British Geriatrics Society, American Academy of Orthopaedic Surgeons algorithm [16].

Despite its utility, this algorithm is not perfect, as up to 20% of individuals deemed *low risk* by the algorithm (i.e., those who have not fallen in the past 12 months) experience a fall in the following year. Moreover, 70% of these falls sustain enough injury to get medical attention [70].

In light of these findings, and based in a recent systematic review of current guidelines in fall prevention [71], we propose a modified approach, summarized in Fig. 3.4.

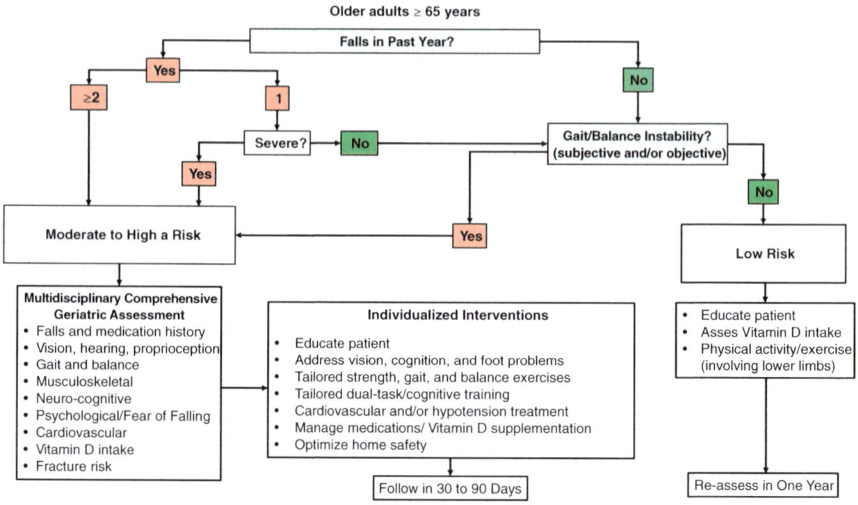

Fig. 3.4 Proposed approach and algorithm to stratify and manage falls in older adults. *Note*: Gait and balance instability: subjective refers to positive answer of feeling unstable while walking, standing, or worries about falling. Objective refers to low performance in a gait/balance test. Severe fall: refers to injury or enough lesions to consult an ER (emergency room)

A comprehensive history of previous falls should be ascertained, as previous falls are a strong predictor of future falls, this is an easy step for commencing the algorithm. A complete and comprehensive fall evaluation for patients who present with a positive history of two falls or one fall with injury during the past year is required as they have an annual incidence of future falls of between 35% and 65%. Specifically, this evaluation should include an assessment of balance and gait, visual acuity, and documentation of the individual's medication history. This triad is considered of high predictive value for detecting older adults at a higher risk of future falls [16]. Next, the individual's basic and instrumental activities of daily living, cognitive abilities, and environmental hazards in the home should be reviewed in detail [72]. Further details on falls assessment in older adults with a history of falls are documented in Table 3.5. All this assessment to detect risk factors is part of the Comprehensive Geriatric Assessment (CGA).

Table 3.5 Cause of falls according to risk factor identification and grouped regarding potential management based on observational studies and clinical trials evidence

Domain assessed	Risk factor/ disease	Level of evidence[a]	Screen/ assessment	Management
Neuromuscular	Parkinsonism syndrome	Ia	Gait velocity test	1. Supervised programs (structural gait retraining, balance, transfer and mobility interventions, progressive limb strengthening and flexibility exercises)
	Balance and gait problems	Ia	Get Up and Go	2. Provision of appropriate walking aids when needed
	Lower extremity weakness	Ia	POMA	3. Vitamin D and calcium supplementation
Medical	Dizziness or vertigo	II	History and examination, including review of drugs, visual acuity assessment, echocardiograph, short Geriatric Depression Scale	1. Appropriate investigation and management of untreated medical problems
	Visual impairment	Ib for cataracts, III for visual acuity		
	Peripheral neuropathy	n/a	CAGE questionnaire	2. Review and modification of psychotropic drugs, other culprit drugs, and polypharmacy. Alcohol counselling if indicated
	Psychoactive medication/ alcohol	Ia		3. Optical correction by an optician or referral to an ophthalmologist
	Hip problems or deformity	n/a		4. Formal psychogeriatric assessment
	Cognitive problems or depression	III		

Table 3.5 (continued)

Domain assessed	Risk factor/ disease	Level of evidence[a]	Screen/ assessment	Management
Environmental	Environmental fall hazards	Ia	Occupational therapy: assessment of environmental fall hazards using a standard checklist	1. Home hazard modification using standard protocol
	Footwear	III		2. Advise to wear well-fitting shoes of low heel height and high surface contact
	Multifocal eyeglasses	II	Check footwear	3. Avoid multifocal eyeglasses while walking
Cardiovascular	Orthostatic hypotension	Ia	Cardiac evaluation including heart rate, morning orthostatic blood pressure, and carotid sinus massage supine and tilted upright, prolonged head-up tilt, if indicated	1. Advice on avoiding precipitants and modification of drugs
	Postprandial hypotension	Ib		2. Postural hypotension: compression hosiery, fludrocortisone, or midodrine
	Vasovagal syndrome	Ia		3. Cardioinhibitory carotid sinus hypersensitivity: permanent pacemaker
	Carotid sinus hypersensitivity	Ib		4. Symptomatic vasodepressor carotid sinus hypersensitivity or vasovagal syncope: fludrocortisone or midodrine

[a]Level of evidence based on reference [83] as following: class Ia, evidence from at least two randomized controlled trials; Ib, evidence from one randomized controlled trial or meta-analysis of randomized controlled trials; II, evidence from at least one nonrandomized controlled trial or quasi-experimental study; III, evidence from prospective cohort study; IV, based on expert committee opinion or clinical experience in absence of other evidence

Because many older individuals who have not already fallen are at increased risk of falling, we strongly suggest conducting a gait and balance evaluation as a screening tool for all older patients as a component of their annual health visits [16, 25, 51, 56, 73].

Gait performance can be assessed in a multitude of ways, with the majority of validated tests in use today being a modification of a test first described by Mathias and Isaacs in 1986, namely the "Get Up and Go Test" [74]. The Get Up and Go Test was initially created to evaluate frail older persons with disabilities; it asks individuals to rise from a chair, walk 3 meters, turn around, walk back to the start point, and sit down. Podsialdo and Richardson (1991) incorporated a timed component to the test [75] and called it, the "Timed Up and Go Test". Individuals at a normal to high functioning level tend to perform well on the task, and therefore a ceiling effect in the timing part of the test tends to occur [76]. Thus, for high functioning individuals, a shorter cut-off time of 12 seconds has been proposed [77]. In addition to modifications of the Get Up and Go Test, more complex tests such as the Performed Oriented

Mobility Assessment (POMA) test and the Berg Balance Scale have been described and validated for assessing risk of falling in various scenarios [78–80].

Simple observational gait evaluations can also be conducted and include the following nine components: (1) initiation of gait, (2) step height, (3) step length, (4) step symmetry, (5) step continuity, (6) path deviation, (7) trunk stability, (8) walking stance, and (9) turning while walking [80]. Each component is scored as a binary variable with 1 for normal observations and 0 for abnormal observations. In simple gait observational evaluations, a total score can be calculated, with higher scores indicating a better gait performance.

Gait speed has also been demonstrated as a strong predictor of falls, even in high functioning older adults. Gait speed is measured as the time taken to walk a known and predetermined distance [56] with the participants being instructed to "walk at a comfortable and secure pace". In situations in which older persons use an assistive device, interpretation of gait speed can be difficult [76]. Thus, gait and balance testing need to be tailored to the population under evaluation. The Get Up and Go Test may be best suited for frail seniors in rehabilitation centers or long-term care settings. Conversely, for higher functioning older adults, gait speed may be a more appropriate tool. Once a gait problem has been detected with a quantitative test, it can be categorized with clinical observation using the hierarchical classification (Table 3.4).

A single test of gait speed may serve as an initial step in a falls risk assessment, with different cut-off points depending on the population being evaluated. As an example, to predict future falls, a gait velocity cut-off of 1 m/s in community living seniors without disability can be used, a cut-off of 0.8 m/s can be used in older persons with disabilities, and a cut-off of 0.6 m/s can be used in older persons living in nursing homes [51, 56, 57]. Dual-task gait testing is most useful in older adults who have a gait speed over 1 m/s or when subtle cognitive impairment is suspected to be contributing to poor motor control.

In addition to gait testing, it is also recommended to perform assessments of the risk of sustaining an injury. Important injury risk factors include a history of a previous osteoporosis fracture, the use of psychotropic medication, the presence of cognitive impairment, sarcopenia, and impaired mobility [81]. This stepped approach to assessment is summarized in Fig. 3.4. Once an assessment is completed and an injury risk categorization has been determined, appropriate, and focused strategies and interventions can be implemented based on global recommendation for those with low risk, with tailored and individualized recommendations for those with moderate and high risk. It has been suggested that those with high risk should have a close follow -up at 30 to 90 days to evaluate the proposed plan or interventions deemed to reduce identified risk factors [82].

Conclusion

In summary, falls are common among older adults and are often accompanied by a plethora of psychological, social, physiological, and medical consequences, even increased mortality. Due to the complexity of contributing factors to a given fall, it is difficult to identify a specific target of falls, and a comprehensive and stepped approach is advocated. Increasing age, hospitalization, and a history of a previous fall are some factors that increase the risk of experiencing a future fall. Additional factors include cognitive deficits, the use of certain medications, and polypharmacy. Although previous falls are predictive of future falls, there is still a considerable number of older individuals who fall despite having no previous falls. In this chapter, we recommend a careful and stepped approach to assess fall risk with gait and balance assessments for all older adults.

Older adults with previous falls need to have a comprehensive evaluation addressing all the potential factors described above. Gait and balance assessments are the domains that will yield more information for falls risk in those without a history of falls. If the patient has a previous history of falls, a comprehensive evaluation is needed. Certain cognitive aspects, including attention and executive function, need to be part of the fall risk evaluation. Although this chapter does not address interventions, the stepped assessment proposed here will detect deficits that can be targeted with multifactorial or single interventions, such as medication modification, and resistance and balance exercises. A logical treatment should emerge that involves a combination of medical, rehabilitative, environmental, and psychosocial interventions.

Acknowledgments I am indebted to Nellie Kamkar, Research Coordinator at the "Gait and Brain Lab," Division of Geriatric Medicine at St. Joseph's Health Care, London, ON, Canada, for her endless assistance in the preparation of the manuscript.

References

1. Rubenstein LZ, Robbins AS, Josephson KR, Schulman BL, Osterweil D. The value of assessing falls in an elderly population. A randomized clinical trial. Ann Intern Med. 1990;113(4):308–16.
2. Tinetti ME. Where is the vision for fall prevention? J Am Geriatr Soc. 2001;49(5):676–7.
3. Wild D, Nayak US, Isaacs B. Description, classification and prevention of falls in old people at home. Rheumatol Rehabil. 1981;20(3):153–9.
4. King MB, Tinetti ME. A multifactorial approach to reducing injurious falls. Clin Geriatr Med. 1996;12(4):745–59.
5. Tinetti ME, Speechley M. Prevention of falls among the elderly. N Engl J Med. 1989;320(16):1055–9.
6. Isaacs B. The giants of geriatrics. The challenge of geriatric medicine. Oxford: Oxford University Press; 1992. p. 1–7.
7. Campbell AJ, Spears GF, Borrie MJ, Fitzgerald JL. Falls, elderly women and the cold. Gerontology. 1988;34(4):205–8.
8. Campbell AJ, Borrie MJ, Spears GF. Risk factors for falls in a community-based prospective study of people 70 years and older. J Gerontol. 1989;44(4):M112–M7.
9. Campbell AJ, Borrie MJ, Spears GF, Jackson SL, Brown JS, Fitzgerald JL. Circumstances and consequences of falls experienced by a community population 70 years and over during a prospective study. Age Ageing. 1990;19(2):136–41.
10. Young SW, Abedzadeh CB, White MW. A fall-prevention program for nursing homes. Nurs Manag. 1989;20(11):80. Y-AA, DD, FF
11. Kerse N, Butler M, Robinson E, Todd M. Fall prevention in residential care: a cluster, randomized, controlled trial. J Am Geriatr Soc. 2004;52(4):524–31.

12. Shaw FE, Bond J, Richardson DA, Dawson P, Steen IN, McKeith IG, et al. Multifactorial intervention after a fall in older people with cognitive impairment and dementia presenting to the accident and emergency department: randomised controlled trial. BMJ. 2003;326(7380):73.
13. Theodos P. Fall prevention in frail elderly nursing home residents: a challenge to case management: part II. Lippincotts Case Manag. 2004;9(1):32–44.
14. Tinetti ME, Baker DI, McAvay G, Claus EB, Garrett P, Gottschalk M, et al. A multifactorial intervention to reduce the risk of falling among elderly people living in the community. N Engl J Med. 1994;331(13):821–7.
15. Tinetti ME, McAvay G, Claus E. Does multiple risk factor reduction explain the reduction in fall rate in the Yale FICSIT trial? Frailty and injuries cooperative studies of intervention techniques. Am J Epidemiol. 1996;144(4):389–99.
16. American Geriatrics Society, British Geriatrics Society, and American Academy of Orthopaedic Surgeons Panel on Falls Prevention. Guideline for the prevention of falls in older persons. J Am Geriatr Soc. 2001;49(5):664–72.
17. Rubenstein LZ, Josephson KR, Osterweil D. Falls and fall prevention in the nursing home. Clin Geriatr Med. 1996;12(4):881–902.
18. Tinetti ME. Clinical practice. Preventing falls in elderly persons. N Engl J Med. 2003;348(1):42–9.
19. Kannus P, Sievanen H, Palvanen M, Jarvinen T, Parkkari J. Prevention of falls and consequent injuries in elderly people. Lancet. 2005;366(9500):1885–93.
20. Muir SW, Gopaul K, Montero Odasso MM. The role of cognitive impairment in fall risk among older adults: a systematic review and meta-analysis. Age Ageing. 2012;41(3):299–308.
21. Kannus P, Leiponen P, Parkkari J, Palvanen M, Jarvinen M. A sideways fall and hip fracture. Bone. 2006;39(2):383–4.
22. Isaacs B. Clinical and laboratory studies of falls in old people. Prospects for prevention. Clin Geriatr Med. 1985;1(3):513–24.
23. Lach HW. Incidence and risk factors for developing fear of falling in older adults. Public Health Nurs. 2005;22(1):45–52.
24. Lach HW. Self-efficacy and fear of falling: in search of complete theory. J Am Geriatr Soc. 2006;54(2):381–2.
25. Bloem BR, Boers I, Cramer M, Westendorp RG, Gerschlager W. Falls in the elderly. I. Identification of risk factors. Wien Klin Wochenschr. 2001;113(10):352–62.
26. Tinetti ME, Doucette J, Claus E, Marottoli R. Risk factors for serious injury during falls by older persons in the community. J Am Geriatr Soc. 1995;43(11):1214–21.
27. Lach HW, Reed AT, Arfken CL, Miller JP, Paige GD, Birge SJ, et al. Falls in the elderly: reliability of a classification system. J Am Geriatr Soc. 1991;39(2):197–202.
28. Tinetti ME, Speechley M, Ginter SF. Risk factors for falls among elderly persons living in the community. N Engl J Med. 1988;319(26):1701–7.
29. Agostini JV, Tinetti ME. Drugs and falls: rethinking the approach to medication risk in older adults. J Am Geriatr Soc. 2002;50(10):1744–5.
30. Leipzig RM, Cumming RG, Tinetti ME. Drugs and falls in older people: a systematic review and meta-analysis: I. Psychotropic drugs. J Am Geriatr Soc. 1999;47(1):30–9.
31. Leipzig RM, Cumming RG, Tinetti ME. Drugs and falls in older people: a systematic review and meta-analysis: II. Cardiac and analgesic drugs. J Am Geriatr Soc. 1999;47(1):40–50.
32. Moden B, Merlo J, Ohlsson H, Rosvall M. Psychotropic drugs and falling accidents among the elderly: a nested case control study in the whole population of Scania, Sweden. J Epidemiol Community Health. 2010;64(5):440–6.
33. Nurminen J, Puustinen J, Piirtola M, Vahlberg T, Kivela SL. Psychotropic drugs and the risk of fractures in old age: a prospective population-based study. BMC Public Health. 2010;10:396.
34. Hanlon JT, Boudreau RM, Roumani YF, Newman AB, Ruby CM, Wright RM, et al. Number and dosage of central nervous system medications on recurrent falls in community elders: the health, aging and body composition study. J Gerontol A Biol Sci Med Sci. 2009;64(4):492–8.
35. Seppala LJ, Wermelink A, de Vries M, Ploegmakers KJ, van de Glind EMM, Daams JG, et al. Fall-risk-increasing drugs: a systematic review and meta-analysis: II. Psychotropics. J Am Med Dir Assoc. 2018;19(4):371 e11–7.

36. Koski K, Luukinen H, Laippala P, Kivela SL. Physiological factors and medications as predictors of injurious falls by elderly people: a prospective population-based study. Age Ageing. 1996;25(1):29–38.
37. Maki BE, McIlroy WE. Postural control in the older adult. Clin Geriatr Med. 1996;12(4):635–58.
38. Maki BE, McIlroy WE. The role of limb movements in maintaining upright stance: the "change-in-support" strategy. Phys Ther. 1997;77(5):488–507.
39. McIlroy WE, Maki BE. Preferred placement of the feet during quiet stance: development of a standardized foot placement for balance testing. Clin Biomech (Bristol, Avon). 1997;12(1):66–70.
40. McIlroy WE, Maki BE. The control of lateral stability during rapid stepping reactions evoked by antero-posterior perturbation: does anticipatory control play a role? Gait Posture. 1999;9(3):190–8.
41. Montero-Odasso M, Hachinski V. Preludes to brain failure: executive dysfunction and gait disturbances. Neurol Sci. 2014;35(4):601–4.
42. Hausdorff JM, Yogev G, Springer S, Simon ES, Giladi N. Walking is more like catching than tapping: gait in the elderly as a complex cognitive task. Exp Brain Res. 2005;164(4):541–8.
43. Yogev-Seligmann G, Hausdorff JM, Giladi N. The role of executive function and attention in gait. Mov Disord. 2008;23(3):329–42.
44. Lundin-Olsson L, Nyberg L, Gustafson Y. "Stops walking when talking" as a predictor of falls in elderly people. Lancet. 1997;349(9052):617.
45. Herman T, Mirelman A, Giladi N, Schweiger A, Hausdorff JM. Executive control deficits as a prodrome to falls in healthy older adults: a prospective study linking thinking, walking, and falling. J Gerontol A Biol Sci Med Sci. 2010;65(10):1086–92.
46. Muir SW, Speechley M, Wells J, Borrie M, Gopaul K, Montero-Odasso M. Gait assessment in mild cognitive impairment and Alzheimer's disease: the effect of dual-task challenges across the cognitive spectrum. Gait Posture. 2011;35(1):96–100.
47. Montero-Odasso M, Bergman H, Phillips NA, Wong CH, Sourial N, Chertkow H. Dual-tasking and gait in people with mild cognitive impairment. The effect of working memory. BMC Geriatr. 2009;9:41.
48. Montero-Odasso M, Muir SW, Speechley M. Dual-task complexity affects gait in people with mild cognitive impairment: the interplay between gait variability, dual tasking, and risk of falls. Arch Phys Med Rehabil. 2012;93(2):293–9.
49. Montero-Odasso M, Wells J, Borrie M. Can cognitive enhancers reduce the risk of falls in people with dementia? An open-label study with controls. J Am Geriatr Soc. 2009;57(2):359–60.
50. Montero-Odasso M, Muir-Hunter SW, Oteng-Amoako A, Gopaul K, Islam A, Borrie M, et al. Donepezil improves gait performance in older adults with mild Alzheimer's disease: a phase II clinical trial. J Alzheimers Dis. 2015;43(1):193–9.
51. Alexander NB. Gait disorders in older adults. J Am Geriatr Soc. 1996;44(4):434–51.
52. Bloem BR, Gussekloo J, Lagaay AM, Remarque EJ, Haan J, Westendorp RG. Idiopathic senile gait disorders are signs of subclinical disease. J Am Geriatr Soc. 2000;48(9):1098–101.
53. Sudarsky L. Geriatrics: gait disorders in the elderly. N Engl J Med. 1990;322(20):1441–6.
54. Dawson-Hughes B, Harris SS, Krall EA, Dallal GE. Effect of calcium and vitamin D supplementation on bone density in men and women 65 years of age or older. N Engl J Med. 1997;337(10):670–6.
55. Dhesi JK, Jackson SH, Bearne LM, Moniz C, Hurley MV, Swift CG, et al. Vitamin D supplementation improves neuromuscular function in older people who fall. Age Ageing. 2004;33(6):589–95.
56. Montero-Odasso M, Schapira M, Varela C, Pitteri C, Soriano ER, Kaplan R, et al. Gait velocity in senior people. An easy test for detecting mobility impairment in community elderly. J Nutr Health Aging. 2004;8(5):340–3.
57. Montero-Odasso M, Schapira M, Soriano ER, Varela M, Kaplan R, Camera LA, et al. Gait velocity as a single predictor of adverse events in healthy seniors aged 75 years and older. J Gerontol A Biol Sci Med Sci. 2005;60(10):1304–9.
58. Nutt JG, Marsden CD, Thompson PD. Human walking and higher-level gait disorders, particularly in the elderly. Neurology. 1993;43(2):268–79.

59. Hough JC, McHenry MP, Kammer LM. Gait disorders in the elderly. Am Fam Physician. 1987;35(6):191–6.
60. Moreland JD, Richardson JA, Goldsmith CH, Clase CM. Muscle weakness and falls in older adults: a systematic review and meta-analysis. J Am Geriatr Soc. 2004;52(7):1121–9.
61. Carey BJ, Potter JF. Cardiovascular causes of falls. Age Ageing. 2001;30(Suppl 4):19–24.
62. Lipsitz LA. Orthostatic hypotension in the elderly. N Engl J Med. 1989;321(14):952–7.
63. Montero-Odasso M, Schapira M, Duque G, Soriano ER, Kaplan R, Camera LA. Gait disorders are associated with non-cardiovascular falls in elderly people: a preliminary study. BMC Geriatr. 2005;5:15.
64. Montero-Odasso M, Verghese J, Beauchet O, Hausdorff JM. Gait and cognition: a complementary approach to understanding brain function and the risk of falling. J Am Geriatr Soc. 2012;60(11):2127–36.
65. Woollacott M, Shumway-Cook A. Attention and the control of posture and gait: a review of an emerging area of research. Gait Posture. 2002;16(1):1–14.
66. Yamada M, Aoyama T, Arai H, Nagai K, Tanaka B, Uemura K, et al. Dual-task walk is a reliable predictor of falls in robust elderly adults. J Am Geriatr Soc. 2011;59(1):163–4.
67. Beauchet O, Annweiler C, Dubost V, Allali G, Kressig RW, Bridenbaugh S, et al. Stops walking when talking: a predictor of falls in older adults? Eur J Neurol. 2009;16(7):786–95.
68. Menant JC, Schoene D, Sarofim M, Lord SR. Single and dual task tests of gait speed are equivalent in the prediction of falls in older people: a systematic review and meta-analysis. Ageing Res Rev. 2014;16:83–104.
69. Muir SW, Speechley M, Borrie M, Montero OM. Fall risk in cognitively impaired older adults: the value of gait assessment under dual task test challenges. Can J Geriatr. 2010;13(1):46.
70. Montero-Odasso M, Kamkar N, Sarquis-Adamson Y, Pieruccini-Faria F, Bray N, Cullen S, et al. Falls risk stratification: when is "low risk" not low risk? J Am Geriatr Soc. 2020; (Conference publication; In press)
71. Montero-Odasso M, Kamkar N, Sarquis-Adamson Y, Speechley M, Masud T. Falls Prevention and Management in Older Adults. A Systematic Review of Clinical Practice Guidelines. PROSPERO [CRD42020173597].
72. Ganz DA, Bao Y, Shekelle PG, Rubenstein LZ. Will my patient fall? JAMA. 2007;297(1):77–86.
73. Perell KL, Nelson A, Goldman RL, Luther SL, Prieto-Lewis N, Rubenstein LZ. Fall risk assessment measures: an analytic review. J Gerontol A Biol Sci Med Sci. 2001;56(12):M761–M6.
74. Mathias S, Nayak US, Isaacs B. Balance in elderly patients: the "get-up and go" test. Arch Phys Med Rehabil. 1986;67(6):387–9.
75. Podsiadlo D, Richardson S. The timed "Up & Go": a test of basic functional mobility for frail elderly persons. J Am Geriatr Soc. 1991;39(2):142–8.
76. Montero-Odasso M. The value of gait velocity test for high-function populations. J Am Geriatr Soc. 2006;54(12):1949–50.
77. Bischoff HA, Stahelin HB, Monsch AU, Iversen MD, Weyh A, von Dechend M, et al. Identifying a cut-off point for normal mobility: a comparison of the timed 'up and go' test in community-dwelling and institutionalised elderly women. Age Ageing. 2003;32(3):315–20.
78. Berg K, Norman KE. Functional assessment of balance and gait. Clin Geriatr Med. 1996;12(4):705–23.
79. Berg KO, Wood-Dauphinee SL, Williams JI, Maki B. Measuring balance in the elderly: validation of an instrument. Can J Public Health. 1992;83(Suppl 2):S7–11.
80. Tinetti ME. Performance-oriented assessment of mobility problems in elderly patients. J Am Geriatr Soc. 1986;34(2):119–26.
81. Gass M, Dawson-Hughes B. Preventing osteoporosis-related fractures: an overview. Am J Med. 2006;119(4 Suppl 1):S3–S11.
82. Stevens JA, Phelan EA. Development of STEADI: a fall prevention resource for health care providers. Health Promot Pract. 2013;14(5):706–14.
83. Tinetti ME, Kumar C. The patient who falls: "It's always a trade-off". JAMA. 2010; 303(3):258–66.

84. Montero-Odasso M. Preventing falls and injuries, and healthy ageing. In: Coll P, editor. Healthy aging a complete guide to clinical management. Cham: Springer International Publishing; 2019.
85. Montero-Odasso M, Speechley M. Falls in cognitively impaired older adults: implications for risk assessment and prevention. J Am Geriatr Soc. 2018;66(2):367–75.

Chapter 4
Immobility Syndrome

Cynthia Irene Mariñansky and José Ricardo Jauregui

Traditional geriatrics focuses on aging-induced functional alterations, which are usually referred to as "Geriatric Giants". One of these "Giants" is the mobility failure, which includes falling, unsteadiness, or simply being stuck in a bed or chair. Mobility problems are important in failing independence, and one could even characterize frailty as failure of cognition, failure of mobility, or both [1–4]. It is very important the interrelation between *immobility syndrome* and the rest of the Geriatric Giants, since immobility can encourage the emergence of the rest of the Giants, while they can induce or accelerate the *immobility syndrome* installation [2, 5]. For example, falls in older people can lead to fractures, which lead to immobility (fracture of column, hip, etc.), but at the same time these falls and fractures can also be favored by the decrease in muscle mass and bone density secondary of a prolonged immobility [6, 7].

Immobility is a common problem which involves a great number of diseases in older individuals, and frequently produce disability, being associated with functional decline, increased risk of nursing home placement after discharge, and medical complications such as deep venous thrombosis, urinary incontinence, pressure sores, joint contractures, cardiac deconditioning, muscle weakness, and falls [2, 7].

Enforced bed rest and immobility are abetted by high beds, intravenous lines and catheters, and both physical (vest, belts, mitten, jacket, and wrist) and chemical restraints that are often used to prevent disruption of treatment and prevent falls. Frequently, they cannot be prevented, but many of its adverse effects may be reduced with simple interventions in order to improve mobility. To enhance patient mobility, physical therapy or graded exercises should be prescribed on the first hospital day, particularly for bed-bound and severely deconditioned patients [7].

C. I. Mariñansky (✉)
Geriatric Division, Durand Hospital, Buenos Aires, Argentina

Maimonides University, Buenos Aires, Argentina

J. R. Jauregui
University of Buenos Aires, Buenos Aires, Argentina

© Springer Nature Switzerland AG 2021

C. G. Musso et al. (eds.), *Frailty and Kidney Disease*,
https://doi.org/10.1007/978-3-030-53529-2_4

The functional evaluation of older individuals has particular importance in those with reduced mobility. It is necessary to determine the basic and instrumental activities of daily life that the individual is able to do by himself, in order to obtain an overview of his situation. It is also highly likely that such activities will worsen in the short term as disable status is maintained [8–10].

It is still certain that the complicated factors involved in clinical mobility problems require the efforts of multiple professionals, as well as a fair amount of time and attention to every detail. The main strategy against the *immobility syndrome* is to avoid or to delay their installation – evolution; for this reason, when the older patient is still able to walk, it is of major importance to perform an evaluation to the patient's posture, march (gait speed, length of the step, etc.), visual-auditive capacity, and environment (lighting, rugs, stairs, etc.) in order to detect, correct, or diminish risk factors for immobility installation [9, 10].

Inactivity was defined as the inability to leave the home oneself at least twice a week. Considering all the non-cardiac risk factors studied, inactivity was found to be the strongest single predictor of death. Preoperative functional deficits contribute to postoperative immobility, associated to complications such as atelectasia and pneumonia, venous stasis and pulmonary embolism, pressure ulcers, and multisystem deconditioning [10, 11].

Untreated or undertreated postoperative pain can have a significant negative impact on the recovery of the older patient following surgery. Pain causes tachycardia, increases myocardial oxygen consumption, and may lead to myocardial ischemia. Because pain is exacerbated by moving, undertreated pain results in immobility, with all the sequel of prolonged bed rest, including pressure ulcers, thromboembolic disorders, and the decline associated with deconditioning [10–12].

Deconditioning, which usually can be traced to excessive bed rest in the home or institution, is a common geriatric phenomenon. It is an important clinical entity characterized by depression and lethargy, anorexia and dehydration, neuromuscular instability, decreased bone density, muscular weakness and incoordination, altered bladder and bowel function with retention and constipation, and urinary and fecal incontinence. Deconditioning leads to further functional decline despite improvement in the acute illness. After surgery, the recovery period of deconditioning can be three or more times longer than the period of immobilization that led to the decline [8, 11].

In the acute hospital, patients should have orders for regular out of bed activities, be encouraged to walk to diagnostic studies if possible, and be taught bed and chair exercises if their mobile capacity is limited. If they do not stress their cardiopulmonary or muscular systems, the presence of deconditioning may go unnoticed [9].

Immobilization can lead to delirium and functional decline within just a few days, yet physicians routinely order bed rest or no activity, often without medical justification [2–4].

Epidemiology and Causes

Immobility increases with age. Eighteen percent of those over 65 have problems moving without help, and after 75 years more than 50% have problems leaving their home, of which 20% are confined to their home. To understand the importance of severe functional impairment of immobilization, it is enough to say that 50% of older individuals who become immobilized in an acute manner die within 6–12 months. Its main causes are as follows [1–5, 13, 14]:

Physical

- Acute illnesses: Urinary tract infections, pneumonia, dehydration, diabetes mellitus complications
- Musculoskeletal disorders: Degenerative joint disease: arthritis, osteoporosis, Paget's disease, hip and femur fractures, podiatric problems such as bunions, calluses, onychomycoses that cause pain and inability to walk
- Neurological disorders: Instability problems, about half the individuals who suffer a stroke have residual deficits for which they require assistance, Parkinson's disease in its later stages, cerebellar dysfunction and neuropathies
- Cardiovascular disease: Severe congestive heart failure, coronary artery disease (frequently with angina), peripheral vascular disease, especially in older diabetics who suffer claudication, which limits ambulation and may result in lower extremity amputations
- Pulmonary disease: Severe chronic obstructive lung disease
- Sensory factors: Impairment of vision

Psychological

- Fear of falling: Especially in those with a history of instability and previous falls, or with impaired vision that can lead to a bed-and-chair existence
- Depression: With its most common manifestation which is decreased mobility

Environmental

- Forced immobility (in hospitals and in nursing homes), inadequate aids for mobility

Iatrogenic Causes

Medication (anti-hypertension drugs, hypnotics, sedatives, neuroleptics). Hospitalization.

Others

- Deconditioning (after extensive bed rest from acute illness)
- Malnutrition
- Severe systemic illness (widespread malignancy).
- Pain

Complications

Prolonged bed rest or inactivity has the following main adverse consequences [2, 5–8, 14–16].

- **Endocrine and metabolic effects**
  Impaired glucose tolerance, diminished plasma volume. Immobilized patients also tend to have lower values of plasma sodium (compared to healthy individuals), and even hyponatremia (natremia <135 mmol/L). This phenomenon has been attributed to a greater retention of free water. Despite this, serum concentrations of other electrolytes, as well as glomerular kidney function are not significantly affected in this syndrome.
- ***Reduction of calcium balance***
  As a consequence of this, bone density is reduced, predisposing it to fractures when the patient is mobilized. In addition, there is an altered body composition (decreased plasma volume), and an altered drug pharmacokinetics.
- ***Psychological* consequences**
  Because of the sensory deprivation, and as they do not receive environmental stimulation, patients often become depressed, deconditioned, and they may present delirium, and seemed to be demented.
- ***Skin and the musculoskeletal system***
  Pressure sores and muscle weakness and atrophy, as well as contractures are frequently observed. Decubitus ulcers, resulting from a protracted prostration, are relatively frequent in the institutional field, although its appearance can be avoided with adequate health care: Pneumatic mattresses, hydro gel in affected areas, patches of support, etc.
- ***Cardiopulmonary complication***
  The combination of deconditioned cardiovascular reflexes and diminished plasma volume can lead to serious postural hypotension, which can impair

rehabilitative efforts. Deep venous thrombosis and pulmonary embolisms are well-known complications. Immobility also impairs pulmonary function: atelectasis may occur, and, when combined with the supine position, it predisposes the development of aspiration pneumonia. The bedridden patient suffers a reduction in ventilatory volume, with an increase in the volume of respiratory secretions. A cough reflex decreased worsens their elimination, favoring the development of serious lung infections (aspiration pneumonia).

- ***Gastrointestinal tract and urine flow are slowed down***
  This predisposes constipation, fecal impaction, the appearance of urinary tract stones and infection. It also produces fecal and urinary incontinence.

The main complications, grouped by importance in the immobilized older patient, are as follows:

Organic complications: Atrophy of the musculature. Contractures and joint ankylosis. Pressure sores. Deep venous thrombosis. Pulmonary embolism. Constipation and fetal impaction. Sphincter incontinence. Sensory deprivation. Cardiorespiratory complications are less frequent than musculoskeletal complications, but the former compromise the patient's life to a greater extent.

Psychological complications: Depressive disorders. Delirium syndrome (psychomotor regressive behavior). Fear of falling

Social complications: Social isolation. Decreased self-esteem. Incapacitation in self-care. Institutionalization

Assessing

The biology of gait and balance ages normally, but the whole system can become deconditioned through disuse and can be damaged by illness or injury. There are several aspects of the medical history and physical examination which are important in the assessment of immobile patients that should be inquired [9, 13]:

- Extent and duration of disabilities causing immobility.
- The underlying medical condition that influences mobility.
- Medications should be reviewed in order to eliminate iatrogenic problems.
- Psychological factors such as depression may cause immobility and be an obstacle to rehabilitation.

- Environment: Inadequate aids for mobility should be modified, and some measures must improve the patient's mobility.
- Physical factors to assess:

  1. The skin: In order to identify early pressure sores.
  2. Cardiopulmonary status: Intravascular volume and postural changes in blood pressure and pulse.
  3. Muscle tone and strength.
  4. Testing of joint range of motion.
  5. Podiatric problems.
  6. Standardized measures of muscle strength can be helpful in gauging a patient's progress.
  7. Hemianopsia, inattention to one side of the body (neglect), and various apraxias are common after strokes.

When comprehensively assessing a frail old person, or anyone who is unsteady, or unable to walk, a specific gait and balance evaluation needs to be added to the usual repertoire. If there is a "mini mental status examination of mobility", it may be the "*get up and go test*": the patient is seated in an armless chair, three meters from a wall. He or she stands, walks,(with walking aids if usually used) towards the wall, turns without touching the wall, returns to the chair, turns, and sits down again. With this test, the physician will know if it is necessary to prescribe walking aids, then by looking at the pattern of movements, he will see if remediable causes of mobility failure are present: pain, Parkinson's disease, vision problems, unsafe footwear, or postural dizziness.

Rehabilitation

It is essential restoring function and preventing further disability in immobile older individuals, and usually requires a team effort. The setting of realistic goals, treatment, and repeated measures of functional abilities that are relevant to the patient's environment are part of the rehabilitation process [14]. Physical therapy in the management of immobile older patients implies to achieve the following objectives:

- Relieve pain.
- Evaluate, maintain, and improve joint range of motion.
- Evaluate and improve strength, endurance, motor skills, and coordination.
- Evaluate and improve gait and stability.
- Assess the need for and teach the use of assistive devices for ambulation (wheelchairs, walkers, canes).

The abovementioned objectives can be achieved through different therapeutic modalities:

- Exercise active and passive
- Heat

- Hydrotherapy
- Ultrasound

General Care

- Prevention of skin problems:
  - The appearance of pressure ulcers is one of the most serious complications in the immobilized patient. To assess patient's risk, you can use the Norton Scale. In this sense, the preventive activities to be carried out are:
- Postural changes:
  - They should follow a certain rotation, always respecting the same posture and body alignment. Make the changes carefully, without dragging the patient, avoiding shear and friction forces. Distribute the body weight equally in order to avoid muscle aches due to compensation contractures.

    In lying patients should be done every 1–2 hours, to minimize the effects of continued pressure on bone prominences.

    In seated patients they will be performed every 10 minutes, lifting it for 10 minutes, to avoid the appearance of pressure ulcers at the sacrum.
- Hygiene:
  - With water and neutral soap and a soft sponge, followed by a good rinse and perfect drying (especially the folds). The bed and/or chair will be clean, dry, and without any foreign objects (breadcrumbs). The sheets should be soft and not wrinkle. The room should be well ventilated and at the right temperature.
- Massage:
  - Activate circulation, promotes muscle relaxation, stimulates sensitivity and facilitates the relationship. It also helps to maintain the body scheme. It should be done gently, gently moving the skin and subcutaneous cellular tissue by wide circular movements (kneading) or pinching and releasing the muscle plane with the fingers again. You can use a moisturizer.
  - Padded in areas of higher pressure, such as elbow, knee, sacrum, trochanters, scapulae, etc.
- Supply of liquids and food:
  - Avoid protein deficits. Recommend an intake of 1–1.5 liters of water per day. A contribution of vitamin C (1 g per day in established ulcers) and Zn (15 mg/day) in the diet is advisable, although the supplements have not been shown to improve healing.
- Prevention of musculoskeletal complications:
  - You should pay attention to posture and body alignment, as well as to perform early movements through active or passive exercises, depending on the patient's situation.

- Prevention of cardiovascular complications:
  It should control blood pressure and heart rate for rhythm disturbances, as well as avoid pulmonary embolisms and phlebitis.
- Prevention of respiratory complications:
  - The stagnation of mucus is a problem to prevent. In order to avoid it, you should follow these recommendations:
    In bedridden patients, it is advisable to keep the head of the bed elevated, perform respiratory physiotherapy, inform the patient that he/she must perform deep inspirations, cough, and expectorate. Sometimes it will be convenient to use aerosols, and it is advisable to drink plenty of liquid to fluidize the secretions and favor their expulsion.
    In the case of poorly collaborated or severely disabled patients, we can establish postural drainage early, whose purpose is the passive elimination of secretions from the specific bronchial area, by placing the patient in postures in which gravity acts. To be effective, these positions must be maintained for 20–30 minutes and repeated a minimum of three times a day. You can also use percussion or clapping, which only has an effect on mass-organized mucus. Percussion should be gentle, taking into account osteoporosis and pain.
- Prevention of gastrointestinal complications:
  - Constipation is a very frequent problem. As a general rule, the diet should be sufficient, balanced, rich in fiber, varied, easily ingested, digested, and absorbed. You should also:
    Check the condition of the mouth (dentition, poorly coupled prostheses, etc.).
    Boost food out of bed and in company to prevent anorexia.
    Incorporate the bedridden patient to avoid bronchoaspiration problems.
    Promote a time pattern of defecation and preserve their privacy.
- Prevention of genitourinary complications:
  - The most pressing problem is incontinence, as well as incomplete bladder emptying, as they will favor urinary infections and stone formation. It is important:
    Maintain an adequate position in urination and privacy conditions.
    If there is incomplete emptying, voluntarily recommend contracting the abdominal wall or exerting manual pressure on it.
    In case of incontinence, perform detrusor training exercises, such as Kegel exercises (start urinating and stop doing so several times during a normal evacuation).
- Prevention of psychological problems:
  - You should favor the expression of feelings and encourage the sharing of emotions.
  - Maintain motivation by setting accessible objectives in the short and medium term. Promote visits and conversation.

Conclusion

Immobility syndrome is one of the main geriatric syndromes, and is tightly related with the rest of them. Hence, older individuals require careful evaluation for this syndrome and the provider should ensure that both its prevention and early treatment are carried out.

References

1. Creditor M. Hazards of hospitalization of the elderly. Ann Intern Med. 1993;118(3):219–23.
2. Forciea M, Lavizzo-Mourey R, et al. Geriatric secrets. Philadelphia: Hanley & Belfus; 2000.
3. Cassel C. et al. Geriatric medicine. An evidence based approach. 4th ed. New York: Springer Science +Business Media, LLC.136, 1115, 274, 242–243.
4. Halter J, Ouslander J, Tinetti M, et al. Hazzard's geriatric medicine and gerontology. New York: The McGraw-Hill Companies; 2009.
5. Hull RD. Relevance of immobility and importance of risk assessment management for medically ill patients. Clin Appl Thromb Hemost. 2013;19(3):268–76.
6. Musso C, Liakopoulos V, Pangre N, DiTrolio J, Jauregui R, De Miguel R, Stefanidis I, Imperiali N, Algranati L. Renal physiology in elderly persons with severe immobility syndrome. Int Urol Nephrol. 2009;41(2):437–41.
7. Reuben DB, et al. Geriatrics at your fingertips: 2016. 18th ed. New York: The American Geriatrics Society; 2016.
8. Shiraki M, Kuroda T, Shiraki Y. Effects of bone mineral density of the lumbar spine and prevalent vertebral fractures on the risk of immobility. Osteoporos Int. 2010;21(9):1545–51.
9. Sloan JP. Protocols in primary care geriatrics/John P. Sloan, 2nd ed. P Libraru of Congress Cataloguing in Publication Data. 1996.33–38.
10. Stall N. Tackling immobility in hospitalized seniors. CMAJ. 2012;184(15):1666–7.
11. Suetta C, Frandsen U, Mackey A. Ageing is associated with diminished muscle re-growth and myogenic precursor cell expansion early after immobility-induced atrophy in human skeletal muscle. J Physiol. 2013;591(15):3789–804.
12. Zarowitz BJ, Tangalos E, Lefkovitz A. Thrombotic risk and immobility in residents of long-term care facilities. J Am Med Dir Assoc. 2010;11(3):211–21.
13. Isaacs B. The challenges of geriatric medicine: Oxford Medical Publications; 1992.
14. Kane R, Ouslander J, Abrass I. Essentials of clinical geriatrics: McGraw-Hill; 1984. p. 153–78.
15. Musso CG, Núñez JF. Feed-back between geriatric syndromes: general system theory in geriatrics. Int Urol Nephrol. 2006;38(3–4):785–6.
16. Reichel W, et al. W.Reichel's care of the Elderl. Clinical aspects of aging. 7th ed. Cambridge/New York: Cambridge University press; 2016. p. 613–7.

Chapter 5
Delirium

Angel Golimstok and Victor Gastón Moreno-Milicich

Introduction

Delirium is a serious acute condition, which consists of a cognitive and behavioral disorder, mainly affecting older people in hospitals. In this disorder, attention, working memory, and consciousness are mainly impaired [1, 2]. Clinically, it is characterized by acute onset and fluctuating course, with behavioral abnormalities (DSM-5) [3].

Delirium is highly prevalent, affecting between 14% and 24% of acute hospital admissions [4], and involves long hospital stay, large health expenses, deterioration of functional performance, cognitive impairment, and increased mortality [5–8]. Three clinical variants have been recognized, one hyperactive, another hypoactive, and a mixed one [9].

The hyperactive variant shows increased motor activity, agitation, anger, or euphoria. In patients with hypoactive delirium, the most prominent findings are decreased motor activity, anxiety, fatigue, amotivational symptoms, and depression [10].

Obviously, the mixed variant is composed of both hyper- and hypoactive symptoms in identical proportion, with difficulty to characterize clinically as one of the two extreme variants. Although many clinicians think that hyperactive delirium is the most frequent, this clinical variant was described representing only 25% of cases [11, 12].

A. Golimstok (✉) · V. G. Moreno-Milicich
Cognition and Behaviour Section, Department of Neurology, Hospital Italiano Buenos Aires, Buenos Aires, Argentina

© Springer Nature Switzerland AG 2021

C. G. Musso et al. (eds.), *Frailty and Kidney Disease*,
https://doi.org/10.1007/978-3-030-53529-2_5

Risk Factors and Triggers for Delirium

Despite delirium having high importance on older individual health and its costs of care, it still remains poorly understood.

In a cohort analytic study performed in 1992, Schor et al. showed [13] independent risk factors for in-hospital delirium. The most important of them was prior cognitive impairment and also included others as fracture on admission, age over 80 years, symptomatic infection, male sex, and both neuroleptic and narcotic use.

Inouye et al. [14] published in 1993 a study of a prospective cohort, identifying four independent baseline risk factors as a higher level of urea/creatinine ratio, cognitive impairment, visual impairment, and severe illness.

A meta-analysis of Ahmed et al. in 2014 [15] identified 11 studies that investigated risk factors for incident delirium in older people with acute medical admission. Ten risk factors statistically associated with incident delirium were found: dementia, comorbid physical illness, severity of physical illness, poor activities of daily living (ADL) function, urinary catheterization, polypharmacy, low albumin, urea/creatinine ratio abnormality (azotemia), low or high sodium, and prolonged hospital stay. Their pooled analysis confirmed statistically significant associations for dementia, illness severity, urinary catheterization, polypharmacy, albumin level, and length of hospital stay. They did not find male gender, depression, and abnormal sodium level as significant risk factors, but this may be due to methodological factors.

In addition to risk factors, it is important to know the delirium triggers. These triggers or precipitants are often multifactorial events. We can classify the triggers in those that occur during hospitalization and those in outpatients.

The former described were the use of physical restraints, malnutrition, polypharmacy, urinary catheter, iatrogenic origin [16], acute renal impairment [17], and psychotropic treatment [18]. The outpatient precipitants were less studied, but infections and falls are the most frequent seen in the daily clinical experience.

The possibility of accurately predicting risk of developing delirium would help to improve preventive measures. In this direction, efforts have been carried out to quantify that presumable risk.

In a recent review of risk-stratification models, the authors found multiple and heterogeneous validated predictive models lacking replication and concluded that further research is needed to support a tool to predict inpatient delirium [19].

Clinical Characteristics of Delirium

Delirium usually begins as an acute or subacute deterioration in behavior, cognition, or general function, with high frequency in older individuals and demented or depressed patients. The patient often develops a change in consciousness with frequent difficulty to focus on environmental stimuli, in a short period of time (in hours). This is particularly evident during the clinical interview. Symptom fluctuation along the day is very often with improvement in the daytime and a peak of alteration at night.

Disturbance of the sleep-wake cycle with insomnia, daytime drowsiness, or disturbing dreams or nightmares can also occur. Patients are generally disoriented in time and space, as well as situationally confused. This disorientation generates false beliefs or thinking, misinterpreting the environment and the actions that surround them. Sometimes the patient with delirium suffers visual and auditory hallucinations, seeing or hearing things that are not present, trying to pick up things in the air, or speaking to somebody who is not there. The aggressive behavior that is frequently seen in these patients is caused by a lack of understanding of their situation, ignoring that they are admitted to the hospital. Delirium in hospitalized patients may result in a fall or injury, self-removal of catheters, or intravenous tubing or bronchoaspiration.

Emotional disturbances are very often, leading to mood impairment, anxiety, fear behavior, and irritability.

Patients may have persecutory delusions as well as grandiose delusions, very frequently, secondary to hallucinations. Some patients are at risk of self- or hetero-aggression. Therefore, they should be monitored very closely. The mental status in these patients consists in most cases of a bedside interview assessment that characteristically fluctuates. Patient's appearance, orientation, short- and long-term memory, mood, behavior symptoms (especially the presence of hallucinations, delusions, and aggressive behavior), and judgment must be evaluated.

In hyperactive variant of delirium, there is an increased state of arousal, psychomotor abnormalities, and hypervigilance. Conversely, in hypoactive delirium, we can find a less active and sleepy patient. Hypoactive delirium sometimes is misdiagnosed as depression.

A subsyndromal delirium with a prevalence of 30–50% in intensive care units has been described as the presence of some core diagnostic symptoms that do not meet the criteria for diagnostic threshold. We should also consider a prodromal phase that can last from a few hours to days before a full syndrome of delirium becomes diagnosable. During this phase, the patient has sleep disturbances, vivid dreams, and anxiety [20, 21].

Diagnosis

The diagnosis is based on clinical features, and we can use DSM-5 diagnostic criteria for delirium [3].

DSM-5 Criteria

(a) Disturbance in attention (i.e., reduced ability to direct, focus, sustain, and shift attention) and awareness (reduced orientation to the environment).

(b) The disturbance develops over a short period of time (usually hours to a few days), represents an acute change from baseline attention and awareness, and tends to fluctuate in severity during the course of a day.
(c) An additional disturbance in cognition (e.g., memory deficit, disorientation, language, visuospatial ability, or perception).
(d) The disturbances in Criteria A and C are not better explained by a preexisting, established, or evolving neurocognitive disorder and do not occur in the context of a severely reduced level of arousal such as coma.
(e) There is evidence from the history, physical examination, or laboratory findings that the disturbance is a direct physiological consequence of another medical condition, substance intoxication or withdrawal (i.e., due to a drug of abuse or to a medication), or exposure to a toxin or is due to multiple etiologies.

A meticulous complete medical history is mandatory, and to assess the patient, a complete physical examination including a mental status examination is necessary.

Impaired attention can be evaluated with bedside tests such as reciting the days of the week or months of the year backwards. The patient can be asked to subtract 7 each time starting at 100.

Other diagnostic instruments are the Delirium Symptom Interview (DSI) and the Confusion Assessment Method (CAM).

Delirium symptom severity can be assessed by the Delirium Rating Scale (DRS) [22].

At the time of admission to the hospital, if the older patient does not have a history of dementia or cognitive impairment, the MoCA is useful to identify patients at high risk for in-hospital delirium [23].

The Confusion Assessment Method for the Intensive Care Unit (CAM-ICU) is suitable to identify delirium in critical care patients, especially patients on mechanical ventilation. The CAM-ICU is based on nonverbal assessments to evaluate the features of delirium [24].

A meta-analysis showed a sensitivity of 75.5% and specificity of 95.8% for CAM-ICU, suggesting that this test is very specific to be used for diagnosing delirium in ICU patients [25, 26].

Laboratory tests are very useful to determine the causes of delirium and rule out other pathologies.

The calcium-binding protein S-100 B could be a potential serum marker of delirium, because a high level of it was described in patients with delirium [27].

Neuroimaging (brain CT scan or MRI) is helpful to rule out other pathologies and determine a structural etiology.

Electroencephalogram should be done when an epilepsy disorder or a prion disease is suspected.

Chest radiograph is used to diagnose pneumonia or congestive heart failure.

Lumbar puncture is needed to diagnose an inflammatory disease in central nervous system (CNS).

Etiology

As we described above, etiology of delirium is multifactorial. Medical disorders, intoxication, or polypharmacy can cause delirium. The potential cause should be clarified in order to find a reversible contributor to the confusional syndrome.

The Most Common Potential Reversible Causes Include the Following

- Hyperthermia
- Hypoxia
- Hypoglycemia /hyperglycemia
- Anticholinergic medications
- Intoxication with alcohol, drugs, or psychotropic medication
- Benzodiazepine withdrawal
- Infections
- Metabolic abnormalities
- Postoperative states
- Urinary retention

Partially Reversible or Not Reversible Causes

- Acute structural lesions of the brain
- Confusional state in dementia
- Stroke
- Craniocerebral trauma
- Vitamin deficiency
- Primary or metastatic brain tumors
- Brain abscess
- Hepatic or renal failure
- Thyroid and parathyroid dysfunction
- Hypertensive encephalopathy
- Encephalitis

Finally, it is interesting to note that underlying dementia is observed in about half of the cases. The presence of dementia increases the risk of delirium two to three times.

Differential Diagnoses

Although according to DSM-5 criteria, it is necessary to exclude delirium in order to diagnose dementia reliably, both entities can be mistaken. In reality, both entities can coexist and this is very frequent as we indicated previously. These syndromes can be clinically differentiated, because the delirium is acute onset, shorter in time, usually reversible, and secondary to some clear precipitating cause. Symptoms of depression are frequent during episodes of delirium, and the hypoactive variant of delirium can be misdiagnosed as depression. Differentiation between both disorders is performed clinically, considering level of consciousness is normal in depression, remembering that up to 42% of patients referred to psychiatry services for suspected depressive illness in the hospital may have delirium.

In addition, delirium may also have to be differentiated from psychotic diseases, but in delirium, there is not usually a previous history of serious psychiatric illness. Furthermore, the onset of symptoms of delirium is acute or subacute, most of hallucinations are visual, and the patient has impairment in level of consciousness.

Delirium Pathophysiology

To date, the delirium pathophysiology is still unclear. As we suggest above, delirium is the result of an interaction of vulnerabilities related to the risk factors, with a trigger or precipitant. This interaction leads to neuroinflammation. When the triggers generate a central insult, as in the case of acute structural lesions of the brain, obviously, neuronal disruption is the consequence. In the case of peripheral triggers, such as urinary retention or an infection, an indirect interaction through peripheral inflammation is generated. Both these mechanisms boost a central inflammatory change with modifications in neurotransmitter action and brain dysfunction.

A recent systematic review analyzed potential rodent models of behavioral and cognitive processes to clarify the pathophysiological processes in delirium.

The authors demonstrated that older individuals and sick rodents develop cognitive and behavior deterioration. The same mechanisms could generate the clinical symptoms of delirium in humans. These symptoms were related to systemic inflammation and a greater production of CNS inflammatory cytokines. The CNS changes observed in systemic inflammation were replicated by administration of various agents including lipopolysaccharide (LPS), SEA, poly I:C, IL-1b, bacterial infection, or multiple types of surgical intervention [28].

In previous reports taken into account by this review, a mild LPS dose injected to both old and younger adult rodents showed an increased IL-6 peripheral inflammatory response in the old group compared to the younger one [29, 30]. Similarly, a clinical study reported in the discussion of that review showed that aged patients that received surgical treatment had higher IL-6 serum levels compared to middle-aged surgical patients [31]. Infection and surgery are the most common precipitants of delirium, and they activated immune cells such as macrophages increasing pro-inflammatory cytokines [32]. These pro-inflammatory cytokines elevated in association with delirium in acute hospitalized patients are IL-6 and IL-8 [33, 34]. The anti-inflammatory cytokine IL-10 was considered to play a role in a potential cytokine imbalance involved in delirium with a negative association with TNFα+IL6 + IL8 [35].

Another proof of the association between delirium and peripheral inflammation is that C-reactive protein (CRP), an acute-phase protein with similar actions to pro-inflammatory cytokines and properties of a marker of peripheral inflammation, raised in its level associated with delirium according to some reports [36, 37].

The association between peripheral inflammation and central inflammation leads to the pathophysiological mechanism called "immune to brain communication" which contributes to understanding of delirium. It is necessary to understand the mechanisms implicated in the link between peripheral and central inflammation. In 2008, Dantzer et al. [38] described the pathways that transduce immune signals from the periphery to the brain.

One of them is the neural pathway, through the activation of primary afferent nerves such as the vagal nerves during abdominal and visceral infections and the trigeminal nerves during oro-lingual infections. Another one is the humoral pathway involving circulating pathogen-associated molecular patterns (PAMPs) that reach the brain at the level of the choroid plexus and the circumventricular organs. PAMPs induce the production and release of pro-inflammatory cytokines by macrophage-like cells expressing Toll-like receptors (TLRs). It is possible to include an increase in blood-brain barrier (BBB) permeability too. This last mechanism is expressed through cytokine release which promotes leucocyte activation and substance release which leads to a subsequent increased BBB permeability.

The delirium biomarker S100β is a cytokine derived from activated glial cells and is a marker of neuronal damage and BBB abnormal permeability. More recently, some reports published higher S100β association with delirium in urinary infections and in hip fracture patients [39, 40]. The microglia activation is the source of neuroinflammation through cytokine release. The delirium precipitants are triggers of neuroinflammation, which induce the microglial cell raise and activation.

The microglial cell activation occurs through Toll-like receptor 4 (TLR4) and the release of pro-inflammatory cytokines [41]. Infections and other causes of delirium interact with TLR4 leading to an increase in released cytokines. Delirium risk factors are responsible for the patient's vulnerability that allows a fertile ground for the above-described mechanisms. These mechanisms are only hypothetical because evidence in humans is lacking and the actual knowledge is based on rodent studies.

Central inflammation mechanisms are less known than peripheral mechanisms in delirium. Postmortem studies in delirium patients showed hippocampal ischemic lesions [42]. An increase of cerebrospinal fluid (CSF) cytokines, a marker of CNS inflammation, was reported as a risk predictor of delirium in the postoperative hip fracture [43].

Delirium in Patients with Chronic Kidney Disease

Delirium is a common cause of morbidity and mortality among patients with chronic kidney disease (CKD). People with end-stage kidney disease (ESKD) are at high risk of delirium as a comorbidity, and it is understandable for the fact that an imbalance in electrolytes, brain adequate nutrients, and hormone alteration are associated with both problems. In addition, chronic renal failure is related to the potential toxic accumulation of substances that can produce delirium. All these failures are more frequent in older individuals receiving multiple medications or suffering from cognitive or behavior impairment and sensory deficit. Patients with renal failure without treatment, inadequate dialysis, transplanted kidney failure, post-dialysis decompensation, infections, and hyperparathyroidism suffer frequently delirium.

Among the types of delirium, there are two most frequent in this group:

1. Uremic encephalopathy. It is a syndrome associated to untreated ESKD. The patients usually show initially lethargy and confusion, with natural progression to seizures and/or coma. Neurologic features are common, such as tremor, myoclonus, or less frequently asterixis. The reversion of the clinical syndrome could be reached with renal replacement treatment.
2. Dialysis decompensation or disequilibrium. It is related to the beginning of the dialysis treatment sessions. Older patients are more vulnerable to this syndrome seen in acute hemodialysis (HD) and even in peritoneal dialysis (PD) and chronic HD. The patients usually present symptoms of headache, nausea, agitation, and sometimes lethargy, seizures, or coma.

Some reports showed that the process of dialysis may contribute to cognitive impairment secondary to large shifts in fluid and urea or through cerebral hypoperfusion and hypoxia with changes in circulating volume [44, 45].

There are very few studies that compare PD and HD consequences on cognitive changes. Some studies suggested advantages of PD over HD, considering that PD induces less frequently hypotension than HD. PD might be associated with better cognitive function secondary to cerebral oxygenation and carotid blood flow, but these findings need more evidence from future studies [46–48].

In patients with CKD, there is a greater susceptibility to delirium associated with cerebrovascular disease, an underlying metabolic and fluid disturbance during dialysis, a high rate of sensory loss, polypharmacy, or increased rate of hospitalization. Potentially toxic metabolites generated by changes in metabolism and clearance of certain drugs may precipitate delirium in patients with CKD. Among the drugs and medications that can produce delirium in CKD, antibiotics, analgesics, and opioids are the most common precipitants [49, 50].

Additionally, acute kidney injury (AKI) was reported to be associated with hyperactive delirium [51], but these results require confirmatory studies.

Treatment

Once the diagnosis of delirium is suspected or confirmed, it is necessary to determine the precipitant of the condition and, if possible, solve it. In the management of this syndrome, there are two types of actions: supportive treatment and pharmacological therapy.

In general terms, the hydration, nutrition, and the metabolic compensation of the patients must be managed by resolving all the internal alterations detected and finally treating his/her symptomatology.

Reality orientation therapy is advisable, but healthcare personnel have the responsibility of providing person-centered and sensitive care to the needs of the older people, remembering that this age group is the one who suffers this disorder more frequently. The environment should be stable, quiet, and well-lighted [52]. Logically, both visual and auditory sensory deficits should be resolved, with the necessary accessories available. Support from a multidisciplinary team should be suggested.

The permanent presence of the caregiver of the patient with delirium during hospitalization is a very important measure to avoid physical restrictions that stress the person and worsen the clinical picture. Another reason to suggest the permanent caregiver presence is to enable permanent reorientation of patient.

Preventive Measures

A patient care program should include the following:

- Ensure that the patients would not be sensory deprived and have the necessary accessories that they usually use.
- Keep the sleep-wakefulness rhythm.
- Prevention of pain.
- Early mobilization.
- Follow-up and treatment of postoperative complications.
- Monitor and help to optimal hydration.
- Provide the necessary nutrition.
- Sphincter control monitoring.

Pharmacological Therapy

In patients with hyperactive delirium with a higher risk of injury to other people or to themselves, treatment with medications should be started. Usually, second-generation antipsychotics medications are useful and better than other strategies [53].

A recent review concluded that benzodiazepines are powerful medications associated with considerable risks and benefits, but they should be used with caution, selecting the right dose, indication, and appropriate timing for the right patient [54].

A pharmacological strategy of increasing use, mainly in patients admitted to ICU, is the administration of low-dose dexmedetomidine. In that sense, a recent publication showed that nocturnal administration of low-dose dexmedetomidine in adults during ICU stay may reduce the incidence of delirium and is associated with better sleep architecture than benzodiazepines [55]. It is desirable that, in the near future, treatment protocols with proven efficacy could be available, for both prevention and palliative care.

Conclusion

Delirium is one of the geriatric giants which have significant importance in older chronic kidney disease patients, particularly in those on renal replacement treatment.

References

1. Fong TG, Tulebaev SR, Inouye SK. Delirium in elderly adults: diagnosis, prevention and treatment. Nat Rev Neurol. 2009;5:210–20.
2. Maclullich AM, Anand A, Davis DH, Jackson T, Barugh AJ, Hall RJ, Ferguson KJ, et al. New horizons in the pathogenesis, assessment and management of delirium. Age Ageing. 2013;42:667–74.
3. American Psychiatric Association. Diagnostic and statistical manual of mental disorders. 5th ed. Washington, DC: American Psychiatric Association; 2013.
4. Inouye SK, Westendorp RGJ, Saczynski JS. Delirium in elderly people. Lancet. 2014;383:911–22.
5. Bellelli G, Morandi A, Di Santo SG, et al. "Delirium Day": a nationwide point prevalence study of delirium in older hospitalized patients using an easy standardized diagnostic tool. BMC Med. 2016;14:106.
6. Davis DH, Muniz Terrera G, Keage H, et al. Delirium is a strong risk factor for dementia in the oldest-old: a population-based cohort study. Brain. 2012;135:2809–16.
7. Guerini F, Frisoni G, Morghen S, et al. Clinical instability as a predictor of negative outcomes among elderly patients admitted to a rehabilitation ward. J Am Med Dir Assoc. 2010;11:443–8.
8. Leslie DL, Marcantonio ER, Zhang Y, et al. One-year health care costs associated with delirium in the elderly population. Arch Intern Med. 2008;168:27–32.
9. Liptzin B, Levkoff SE. An empirical study of delirium subtypes. Br J Psychiatry. 1992;161:843–5.
10. Bourgeois JA, Seritan SA. Diagnosis and management of delirium. Continuum. 2006;12(18): 15–32.
11. Marcantonio ER. In the clinic: delirium. Ann Intern Med. 2011;154(11):ITC6–1.
12. Marcantonio ER. Postoperative delirium: a 76-year-old woman with delirium following surgery. JAMA. 2012;308:73–81.
13. Schor JD, Levkoff SE, Lipsitz LA, Reilly CH, Cleary PD, Rowe JW, Evans DA. Risk factors for delirium in hospitalized elderly. JAMA. 1992;267(6):827–31.

14. Inouye SK, Viscoli CM, Horwitz RI, Hurst LD, Tinetti ME. A predictive model for delirium in hospitalized elderly medical patients based on admission characteristics. Ann Intern Med. 1993;119:474–81.
15. Ahmed S, Leurent B, Sampson EL. Risk factors for incident delirium among older people in acute hospital medical units: a systematic review and meta-analysis. Age Ageing. 2014;43(3):326–33. https://doi.org/10.1093/ageing/afu022. Epub 2014 Mar 6
16. Inouye SK, Charpentier PA. Precipitating factors for delirium in hospitalized elderly persons. Predictive model and interrelationship with baseline vulnerability. JAMA. 1996;275:852–7.
17. O'keeffe ST, Lavan JN. Predicting delirium in elderly patients: development and validation of a risk-stratification model. Age Ageing. 1996;25:317–21.
18. Martinez JA, Belastegui A, Basabe I, Goicoechea X, Aguirre C, Lizeaga N, Urreta I, et al. Derivation and validation of a clinical prediction rule for delirium in patients admitted to a medical ward: an observational study. BMJ Open. 2012;2(5):e001599.
19. Newman MW, et al. Predicting delirium: a review of risk-stratification models. Gen Hosp Psychiatry. 2015; https://doi.org/10.1016/j.genhosppsych.2015.05.003.
20. Cole M, McCusker J, Dendukuri N, Han L. The prognostic significance of subsyndromal delirium in elderly medical inpatients. J Am Geriatr Soc. 2003 Jun.;51(6):754–60.
21. Ouimet S, Riker R, Bergeron N, Cossette M, Kavanagh B, Skrobik Y. Subsyndromal delirium in the ICU: evidence for a disease spectrum. Intensive Care Med. 2007;33(6):1007–13.
22. Paula T, Trzepacz MD, Dinesh Mittal MD, Rafael Torres MD, Kim Kanary BS, John Norton MD, Nita Jimerson MSN. Validation of the delirium rating scale-revised-98: comparison with the delirium rating scale and the cognitive test for delirium. J Neuropsychiatry Clin Neurosci. 2001;13:229–42.
23. Saczynski JS, Inouye SK, Guess J, et al. The Montreal cognitive assessment: creating a crosswalk with the mini-mental state examination. J Am Geriatr Soc. 2015;63(11):2370–4. https://doi.org/10.1111/jgs.13710.
24. Ely EW, Margolin R, Francis J, May L, Truman B, Dittus R, et al. Evaluation of delirium in critically ill patients: validation of the Confusion Assessment Method for the Intensive Care Unit (CAMICU). Crit Care Med. 2001;29:1370–9.
25. Neto AS, Nassar AP Jr, Cardoso SO, Manetta JA, Pereira VG, Espósito DC, et al. Delirium screening in critically ill patients: a systematic review and meta-analysis. Crit Care Med. 2012;40(6):1946–51.
26. Farrell KR, Ganzini L. Misdiagnosing delirium as depression in medically ill elderly patients. Arch Intern Med. 1995;155(22):2459–64.
27. Van Muster BC, Korevaar JC, Korse CM, Bonfer JM, Zwinderman AH, DeRooji SE. Serum S100B in elderly patients with and without delirium. Int J Geriatr Psychiatry. 2010;25(3):234–9.
28. Schreuder L, Eggen BJ, Biber K, Schoemaker RG, Laman JD, de Rooij SE. Pathophysiological and behavioral effects of systemic inflammation in aged and diseased rodents with relevance to delirium: a systematic review. Brain Behav Immun. 2017;62:362–81. https://doi.org/10.1016/j.bbi.2017.01.010.
29. Godbout J, Moreau M, Lestage J, et al. Aging exacerbates depressive-like behavior in mice in response to activation of the peripheral innate immune system. Neuropsychopharmacology. 2008;33:2341–51. https://doi.org/10.1038/sj.npp.1301649.
30. Berg BM, Godbout JP, Chen J, Kelley KW, Johnson RW. α-tocopherol and selenium facilitate recovery from lipopolysaccharide-induced sickness in aged y from lipopolysaccharide-induced sickness in aged mice. J Nutr. 2005;135(5):1157–63. https://doi.org/10.1093/jn/135.5.1157.
31. Thaeter M, Knobe M, Vande Kerckhove M, et al. Eur J Trauma Emerg Surg. 2016;42:547. https://doi.org/10.1007/s00068-016-0719-9.
32. Barton GM. A calculated response: control of inflammation by the innate immune system. J Clin Invest. 2008;118:413–20.
33. de Rooija SE, van Munsterab BC, Korevaarb JC, Levia M. Cytokines and acute phase response in delirium. J Psychosom Res. 2007;62(5):521–5.

34. Egberts A, Wijnbeld EH, Fekkes D, van der Ploeg MA, Ziere G, Hooijkaas H, van der Cammen TJ. Mattace-Raso F Neopterin: a potential biomarker for delirium in elderly patients. Dement Geriatr Cogn Disord. 2015;39(1–2):116–24. https://doi.org/10.1159/000366410. Epub 2014 Nov 19
35. Cerejeira J, Nogueira V, Luís P, Vaz-Serra A, Mukaetova-Ladinska EB. The cholinergic system and inflammation: common pathways in delirium pathophysiology. J Am Geriatr Soc. 2012;60(4):669–75. https://doi.org/10.1111/j.1532-5415.2011.03883.x. Epub 2012 Feb 8
36. White S, Eeles E, O'mahony S, Bayer A. Delirium and C-reactive protein. Age Ageing. 2008;37:123–4; author reply 124
37. Ritchie CW, Newman TH, Leurent B, Sampson EL. The association between C-reactive protein and delirium in 710 acute elderly hospital admissions. Int Psychogeriatr. 2014;26:717–24.
38. Dantzer R, O'connor JC, Freund GG, Johnson RW, Kelley KW. From inflammation to sickness and depression: when the immune system subjugates the brain. Nat Rev Neurosci. 2008;9:46–56.
39. Khan BA, Farber MO, Campbell N, Perkins A, Prasad NK, Hui SL, Miller DK, et al. S100 calcium binding protein B as a biomarker of delirium duration in the intensive care unit – an exploratory analysis. Int J Gen Med. 2013;6:855–61.
40. Hall RJ, Ferguson KJ, Andrews M, Green AJ, White TO, Armstrong IR, Maclullich AM. Delirium and cerebrospinal fluid S100B in hip fracture patients: a preliminary study. Am J Geriatr Psychiatr. 2013;21:1239–43.
41. Jalleh R, Koh K, Choi B, Liu E, Maddison J, Hutchinson MR. Role of microglia and toll-like receptor 4 in the pathophysiology of delirium. Med Hypotheses. 2012;79:735–9.
42. Janz DR, Abel TW, Jackson JC, Gunther ML, Heckers S, Ely EW. Brain autopsy findings in intensive care unit patients previously suffering from delirium: a pilot study. J Crit Care. 2010;25(538):e7–12.
43. Cape E, Hall RJ, Van Munster BC, De Vries A, Howie SE, Pearson A, Middleton SD, et al. Cerebrospinal fluid markers of neuroinflammation in delirium: a role for interleukin-1beta in delirium after hip fracture. J Psychosom Res. 2014;77:219–25.
44. Prohovnik I, et al. Cerebrovascular effects of hemodialysis in chronic kidney disease. J Cereb Blood Flow Metab. 2007;27:1861–9.
45. Patel N, Dalal P, Panesar M. Dialysis disequilibrium syndrome: a narrative review. Semin Dial. 2008;21:493–8.
46. Toyoda K, et al. Stroke in patients on maintenance hemodialysis: a 22-year single- center study. Am J Kidney Dis. 2005;45:1058–66.
47. Tilki HE, Akpolat T, Tunali G, Kara A, Onar MK. Effects of haemodialysis and continuous ambulatory peritoneal dialysis on P300 cognitive potentials in uraemic patients. Ups J Med Sci. 2004;109:43–8.
48. Buoncristiani U, et al. Better preservation of cognitive faculty in continuous ambulatory peritoneal dialysis. Perit Dial Int. 1993;13(Suppl. 2):S202–5.
49. Dean M. Opioids in renal failure and dialysis patients. J Pain Symptom Manag. 2004;28:497–504.
50. Grill MF, Maganti R. Cephalosporin-induced neurotoxicity: clinical manifestations, potential pathogenic mechanisms, and the role of electroencephalographic monitoring. Ann Pharmacother. 2008;42:1843–50.
51. Wan R, McKenzie CA, Taylor D, Camporota L, Ostermann M. Acute kidney injury as a risk factor of hyperactive delirium: a case control study. J Crit Care. 2020;55:194–7.
52. Day J, Higgins I, Keatinge D. Orientation strategies during delirium: are they helpful? J Clin Nurs. 2011;20(23–24):3285–94. https://doi.org/10.1111/j.1365-2702.2011.03849.x. Epub 2011 Sep 21
53. Kishi T, Hirota T, Matsunaga S, Iwata N. Antipsychotic medications for the treatment of delirium: a systematic review and meta-analysis of randomised controlled trials. J Neurol Neurosurg Psychiatry. 2016;87(7):767–74. https://doi.org/10.1136/jnnp-2015-311049. Epub 2015 Sep 4

54. Hui D. Benzodiazepines for agitation in patients with delirium: selecting the right patient, right time, and right indication. 1. Curr Opin Support Palliat Care. 2018 Dec;12(4):489–94. https://doi.org/10.1097/SPC.0000000000000395.
55. Skrobik Y, Duprey MS, Hill NS, Devlin JW. Low-Dose Nocturnal Dexmedetomidine Prevents ICU Delirium. A Randomized, Placebo-controlled Trial. Am J Respir Crit Care Med. 2018;197(9):1147–56. https://doi.org/10.1164/rccm.201710-1995OC.

Chapter 6
Urinary Incontinence in Older Persons

José Ricardo Jauregui

Introduction

Urinary incontinence (UI) is considered one of the most frequent chronic problems in outpatients with maximum expression in older individuals; being even more prevalent than diabetes mellitus or Alzheimer's disease. With the aging population of developed or developing countries, the expenditure of health systems in problems generated by the UI quadrupled in relation to the previous decade. As the older population in the world began to increase, UI became more frequent, but it was considered a problem of nursing management and general care or a sign that accompanied the aging process. Although it is true that there are physiological changes that favor the appearance of UI, this is not a "normal" problem of old age. Despite its high prevalence, this is an underdiagnosed and subtracted issue, and the diffusion of this disabling alteration is far from satisfactory, this is the first obstacle, although not the only one for patients to access appropriate treatment (Fig. 6.1).

Explicit conversation about this problem should be part of the functional evaluation of older patients.

The embarrassment of having UI drives most patients to not seek a solution. Only between 13% and 51% of women have talked to their doctor about the issue, but not as part of the central reason for the consultation, or have made an appointment specifically for the problem. A study conducted with ambulatory older individuals covered by the health plan of the Hospital Italiano de Buenos Aires, showed that out of the group of patients with UI, only 7% of them reported that their family

J. R. Jauregui (✉)
University of Buenos Aires, Buenos Aires, Argentina

© Springer Nature Switzerland AG 2021

C. G. Musso et al. (eds.), *Frailty and Kidney Disease*,
https://doi.org/10.1007/978-3-030-53529-2_6

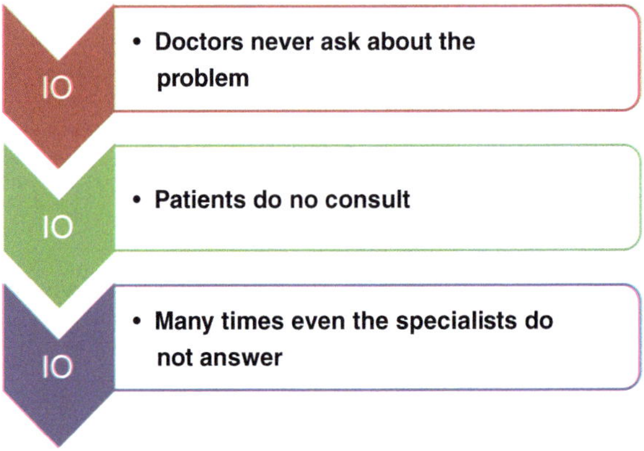

Fig. 6.1 Barriers for detection and treatment of Urinary Incontinence

doctors knew the problem. It is interesting to point out that most of the specialists do not give answers to this "occasional" consultation; sometimes due to discomfort, and others because it is considered part of the normal ageing process. Similarly, patients do not mention this problem because they believe that it has no solution, or that the available ones require them to undergo complicated studies or treatments [1].

However, it should be clear that UI in older persons is always a pathological process, since the changes that normally are associated with physiological aging can predispose but never justify the problem.

Definition

There are many definitions in the literature, but the one proposed by the International Continence Society (ICS) states the following:

Incontinence is the involuntary and objectoniable loss of urine through the intact urethra, severe enough to cause hygienic and social consequences.

In 2002 the ICS changed that definition to that of "involuntary and objective loss of urine through the intact urethra", making it more inclusive so that even without having hygienic and social consequences, it is still a health problem; leading to more cases being diagnosed. It is also said that a patient is incontinent when the urine loss occurres more than once in the last month or more than twice in the last year.

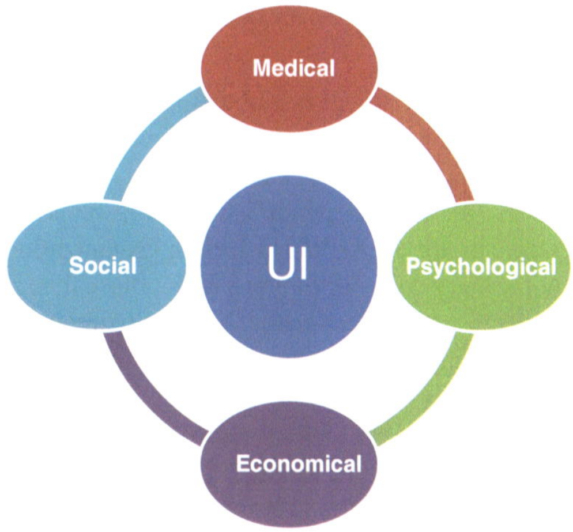

Fig. 6.2 Consequencies of Urinary Incontinence

Relevance of the Problem

It is important to keep in mind that the relevance of UI is not only due to its high prevalence but also due to the complications that this problem can potentially generate (Fig. 6.2).

> The UI has an impact on the quality of individual life and the relationship of the people who suffer it.

UI is associated with a large number of medical problems. Such as urinary tract infections, pressure ulcers, skin irritation, bedsores, falls, and, subsequently, fractures. From a psychological point of view, the consequences can be devastating, with an impact on work activity and social participation. These limitations affect the social life of those people who suffer from UI, and can lead to situations of anxiety, anguish, depression, dependence, confusion, and isolation. Usually patients tend to organize their life around the problem. UI also causes economic consequences that include expenses related to illness, such as medication, special care, dressings, diapers and disposable materials, and those related to other medical complications without counting the cost of the losses in quality of life. This cost has an impact not only on the individual level, but also on the family and social levels.

Demographic Aspects and Epidemiology of the UI

The prevalence of UI in ambulatory and autonomous population older than 65 years is between 15% and 25%, with predominance in women; in special populations, such as older individuals hospitalized for an acute problem, the institutionalized, or the insane, UI prevalence increases progressively to 33%, 50%, and 90%, respectively. In 1998, the World Health Organization (WHO) presented a report stating that urinary control problems affect more than 200 million people worldwide. In the United States, an estimated 700,000 women suffer from this disease. In 2004, a US study (conducted by the National Association for Continence) stated that, after starting UI symptoms, women wait 6.5 years and men 4.2 years before reaching a doctor. In 2004 another study done in Spain by the "National Incontinence Observatory Group," found that the global UI prevalence was of 23% [2–15].

In conclusion, the prevalence of UI increases with age, becoming highly prevalent in people over 65 years of age, especially in women over 80 years old (in some countries over 40%). This causes a high impact on the people's health and quality of life, which forces health agents to be attentive to their appearance, consequences, and treatments that can be offered [3].

Anatomy and Physiology of the Urinary Tract

In a practical way, three definite structures are involved in urination and urine continence:

The structures described in Fig. 6.3 are under delicate control of the autonomic nervous system and the central nervous system. In addition to these structures of the urinary tree, we must take into account the extrinsic urethral component of urinary continence. It is vital to understand the role of this component in patients' urinary continence rehabilitation. Normally, the pelvic floor has an elasticity that allows, when tensed by the pubococcygeal muscles, to hold the urethra inside the

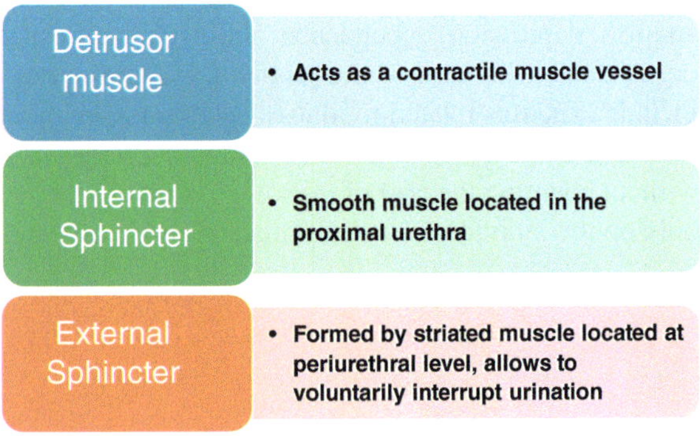

Fig. 6.3 Structures that participate in urination and continence

abdominal cavity, which closes the vesicourethral angle and contributes to urinary continence during the increase of the intra-abdominal pressure. The nervous system interactions are organized into four levels to control urination: the first and the second control detrusor innervation, while the third and fourth modulate the periurethral innervation and striated muscle of the urethral sphincter.

- **Level 1:** It is formed by descending axons, which connect the cortex of the frontal lobe and the thalamus with the detrusor nucleus in the brainstem (pontine nucleus). This level has an inhibitory effect on the detrusor nucleus in the trunk, located between the bridge and the cerebellum (normally the detrusor contracts when receiving the stimulus coming from the trunk nucleus). The detrusor remains relaxed while level 1 exerts its inhibitory effect on this nucleus and contracts when the inhibitory effect disappears voluntarily, which frees the nucleus from the trunk and stimulates detrusor contraction.
- **Level 2**: It is formed by sensory axons that go from the bladder to the sacral spine, through the pelvic nerves. From there, they ascend without synapses to the pontine nucleus of the detrusor. This route informs the pontine center that the detrusor has started a reflex contraction. Impulses generated from this nucleus descend to the motor nucleus of the detrusor, located in the medullary cone. The motor neurons of the medullary cone send axons to the roots S2, S3, and S4, with synapses in the peripheral pelvic ganglion (hypogastric plexus), from which the postganglionic axons further stimulate the detrusor's contraction and reinforce the contraction that had begun in reflex form. This level forms the primary reflex arc of the detrusor innervation.
- **Level 3**: It is constituted by proprioceptive fibers originating in the detrusor that travel through the pudendal nerves and their nuclei in the medullary cone. These sensory impulses inhibit the tonic motor impulses, which normally maintain the tone of the pelvic floor musculature. The net effect of this level is to produce passive relaxation of the pelvic floor muscles during bladder filling.
- **Level 4**: It is formed by the affections of the neuromuscular spindle of the striated muscle of the urethral sphincter, the anal sphincter, and the pelvic floor musculature. These afferents pass through the posterior cords of the spinal cord to end in the cerebellum, thalamus, and sensory-motor cortex of the frontal lobe. The response goes down through the cortex-spinal beam to the motor neurons located in the pudendal nuclei. This level facilitates the voluntary control of urination. The pelvic nodes receive motor impulses from the lumbosacral spine and send postganglionic fibers to innervate the detrusor. The pelvic nodes respond individually to the sympathetic and parasympathetic innervations; usually the sympathetic stimulation inhibits the parasympathetic impulses and vice versa.

To summarise the net effect of the interaction of the nuclei of the nervous system with the pelvic nodes is to communicate the bladder filling state to the brain.

When the maximum state of bladder distension is reached, detrusor contraction (facilitated by level 2) and bladder emptying occur. This reflex response can be inhibited voluntarily by the effect of superior cortical control on the lower nuclei (level 1). When the person finds a suitable place and time to urinate, the inhibition of the central nervous system (CNS) is interrupted, and the contractions (stimulated from level 2) initiate the bladder emptying (Level 4). These contractions are compounded by the effect of increased intra-abdominal pressure through the contractions of the pelvic floor muscles. Finally, this circuit is synchronized with the relaxation of the bladder outlet tract and urethral sphincter (levels 3 and 4). The localization of autonomic neuroreceptors has made it possible to advance in the understanding of the complete organization of the lower urinary tract. The α-adrenergic sympathetic receptors predominate in the bladder outlet cone and along the urethra and are responsible for the maintenance of continence due to increased urethral tone. The sympathetic β-adrenergic receptors are located mainly in the body and vesical dome. The stimulation of these receptors allows the relaxation of the detrusor and the filling of the bladder. That is, the sympathetic impulses favor bladder filling since they relax the bladder and contract the urethral sphincter and the bladder neck. Most parasympathetic (cholinergic) receptors are found in the bladder, but are also located in the bladder outlet cone and along the urethra. The stimulation of these receptors causes the contraction of the detrusor and, as a consequence, the onset of urination.

Continence and urination occur as a consequence of a delicate mechanism in which the autonomic nervous system participates. The sympathetic stimulation favors bladder filling since it relaxes the bladder and contracts the urethral sphincter and the bladder neck. The parasympathetic stimulation favors bladder emptying due to detrusor contraction and simultaneous inhibition of sympathetic activity. This system of reflex action is under voluntary cortical control.

Changes of the Genitourinary System Associated with Normal Aging

During normal aging, there are certain changes in the lower urinary tract which, added to the decrease in the mobility of the older individuals, predispose but do not determine the appearance of UI. The feeling of full bladder in older individuals appears only at 500–600 ml, while in young people it appears at 400 ml. Decreases the ability to postpone bladder emptying. In women, the maximum closing pressure of the external sphincter is reduced. The 25 ml postvoid residue in young people increases to 100 ml in the older individual because the bladder does not discharge its volume completely due to a decrease in the contractile force of the detrusor. The micturition frequency pattern is modified, being more frequent at night. In the oldest individuals (older than 75 years), the size of the brain (atrophy) decreases as part of normal aging, so the trunk nuclei responsible for inhibiting detrusor contractions loses strength, and as inhibition weakens, the contractions are stronger and followed, and the urge to urinate suddenly appears due to an increase in detrusor contractions. The rapid decline of the ovaries is one of the physiological changes mostly related to aging in women, marking the beginning of their menopause. At menopause, ovarian estrogen production is markedly diminished or nonexistent. After menopause, the secretion of progesterone drops markedly. The atrophic changes in the uterus and vagina are caused by the low level of estrogen. In the vagina, the epithelium becomes thinner, the vaginal secretions decrease, pH increases and there is a fall of the trophism of all the urogenital tissue. Consequently, this alters the normal vaginal microbial flora, which is easily colonized by the anal margin, favoring urinary infections. To conclude, there is atrophy of the entire urogenital apparatus accompanied by a fall in functionality, which is manifested by the decrease in secretions and the thinning of the urogenital tissue.

The changes produced in the urinary tract are marked and represent a condition that favors the appearance of urinary incontinence associated with age due to its weakness or atrophy.

The pelvic floor muscles are weakened due to the previously described changes, in addition to muscular atrophy due to disuse or sarcopenia, the possible history of multiparity on woman and a lack of physical exercise or obesity, muscle fibers are thinned or replaced by connective tissue. All this prevents the pelvic floor from contracting and stiffening during urination. Thus, it does not support the neck of the urethra and causes urethral hypermobility with lack of occlusion of the vesicourethral angle. The atrophy of this muscle group is the main cause of stress incontinence on older woman. We should remember that the detrusor muscle responds just like the myocardium, contracting when it undergoes stretching (Frank Starling). This means that distention or bladder filling will produce involuntary muscle contractions if not inhibited. The aging process of the central nervous system, mainly of the frontal cortex, affects the function of the urination control nuclei. These nuclei are under superior inhibition, which ceases with a decreased frontal cortex function due to aging. As a result, a sense of urgency appears, which is called bladder not inhibited or overactive (Table 6.1).

Pathophysiology of Urinary Incontinence

Normal function of the lower urinary tract requires the ability to accumulate urine within the bladder, at low pressure and with the detrusor at rest, as well as the ability to voluntarily complete bladder emptying through a urethra that generates low resistance to emptying. From the above, it follows that for this function to be normal, it is necessary that both the detrusor muscle and the urethra function properly, without forgetting that for the whole process to be performed in a normal manner, these organs must have a normal relationship with the muscles of the body, pelvic floor,

Table 6.1 Urinary incontinence secondary to aging

Changes related to aging	Potential effects
Detrusor degeneration	Altered bladder contractility
Disunion pattern in electron microscopy	Detrusor overactivity
Alteration of the cellular function	Alteration of mucous membranes and connective tissue
Hypoestrogenemia	Thinner and friable fabrics (membranes)
	Increased risk of urinary symptoms, prolapse, and infections
Alteration in the concentration of neurotransmitters	Increased risk of bladder and urethral dysfunction
Impaired immune function	Greater susceptibility to infection
Alteration of bladder function	Increased risk of urinary symptoms, incontinence, and infections
Involuntary contractions	
Decrease in contractility	
Higher residual volume	
Decreased urethral pressure	Increased risk of incontinence

Table 6.2 Requirements for the maintenance of urinary continence in older individuals

Adequate storage in the lower urinary tract
Adequate voiding of the lower urinary tract
Enough motivation to be continent
Enough cognitive capacity to perceive micturition desire
Mobility and sufficient skill to reach the bathroom
No environmental barriers that limit access to the bathroom

fascias, and ligaments that support them and the neural elements that govern both the intrinsic urinary function and the extrinsic elements above mentioned (Table 6.2).

Stress Urinary Incontinence (SUI)

Although pregnancy, vaginal delivery, and the aging processes are the most important determinants for the genesis of stress urine incontinence (SUI), the mechanisms involved in its development are not very clear. During vaginal delivery, there is a disruption of the pelvic anchors of the vagina, together with traction and crushing of the pudendal nerve, stretching of the cardinal and uterosacral ligaments, as well as avulsion of the levator ani muscles. All of this leads to the widening of the genital hiatus and the impoverishment of the support of the pelvic organs. These alterations are repeated with successive deliveries and the injury is cumulative, although the most important damage is done in the first pregnancy. This process leads to a loss of support of the proximal urethra, which undergoes descent and rotation from its retropubic position, generating an alteration known as urethral hypermobility. In this way, when the abdominal pressure increases in a woman with a weakened pelvic floor, the urethra descends beyond normal, and the pressure is transmitted unevenly to the bladder and urethra, with the consequent higher bladder load that leads to urethra incontinence. The loss of the estrogenic stimulus, the denervation of the pelvic floor and the urethral complex, as well as the decrease in the amount of support collagen or its deterioration generate a decrease in the coaptation capacity of the urethra and lead to the symptoms of incontinence. While gestation and vaginal birth can collaborate with this second mechanism, it is more common to find it due to non-obstetric causes, the main one being aging, frequently associated with diseases such as obesity and chronic constipation. In this way, stress urinary incontinence would basically occur due to two conditions: the presence of urethral hypermobility and the inability of intrinsic coaptation of the urethra.

Urgent Urinary Incontinence (UUI)

The term overactive bladder refers to a group of symptoms that include urgency, frequency, and nocturia, associated or not with incontinence. When incontinence is present, it is called urge incontinence. This urgency may or may not be associated with demonstrable non-inhibited bladder contractions due to urodynamics. The basic conflict is constituted by the loss of bladder accommodation capacity, of neurological origin or not. In this second group, the aging process takes on special interest, since most of the overactive bladder syndromes of the postmenopause are constituted by what was once called sensory urgency, that is to say urgency and urinary frequency not associated with the development of contractions. The detrusor inhibitors in urodynamics have fundamental therapeutic implications, since the use of potent anticholinergics is unnecessary in this group of patients that in some series represent up to 70% of cases. In contrast, the use of these drugs is of great help in the group in which bladder contractions are verified. Finally, there are certain pathologies related to urinary incontinence, which can be summarized in Table 6.3.

Classification

In a practical way, the UI can be classified as acute or chronic.

Acute Urinary Incontinence

It is called acute urinary incontinence to any episode that occurred in the 6 months prior to the consultation, in an acute form, and that has responded to the imposed treatments.

The most frequent causes are recorded in the word mnemonic "Diappers":

- D (Delirium)
- I (Infection: urinary infection due to local irritation within the framework of delirium)

Table 6.3 Frequent pathologies in elderly people with continence impact

Pathologies	Mechanisms
Cognitive and sensory impairment	Decreased ability to report symptoms
Motor disorders and immobility	Difficulty to get to the bathroom. Increased risk of incontinence
Stroke	
Hip fracture	
Parkinson's disease	
Peripheral vascular disease	
Low intake of liquids	Increased risk of bacteriuria
Diuretic intake	Polyuria that predisposes to incontinence
Alcohol	
Caffeine	
Diabetes mellitus	Polyuria that predisposes to incontinence
Volume overload	Higher night risk
Heart failure	
Venous insufficiency	
Medication	Increased risk of bladder or urethral dysfunction
Tumors	Increased risk of bladder or urethral dysfunction
Arteriosclerosis	Increased risk of bladder or urethral dysfunction

Table 6.4 UI caused by drugs

Type of medication	Potential effect
Diuretics	Polyuria, frequency increase, urgency
Anticholinergic	Urinary retention, UI overflow
Antidepressants	Anticholinergic effect, sedation
Antipsychotics	Anticholinergic effect, sedation, rigidity, immobility
Sedative hypnotics	Sedation, delirium, immobility, muscle relaxation
Lithium	Polyuria, frequency, urgency
Opioids	Urinary retention, sedation, delirium
α-Blockers	Urinary retention
α-Agonists	Urinary retention
β-Agonists	Urinary retention
Calcium channel blockers	Urinary retention
ACEIs	Chronic cough favors UI
Alcohol	Polyuria, sedation

ACEIs angiotensin-converting enzyme inhibitors

- A (Atrophic: vaginitis or urethritis. Changes local pH and promotes bacterial development)
- P (Pharmaceuticals: drugs) (Table 6.4)
- P (Psychological: depression, dementia, isolation)
- E (Endocrinopathy, such as hyperglycemia, hypercalcemia, hypokalemia)
- R (Restriction of mobility. Functional UI)
- S (Stool impaction)

Chronic Urinary Incontinence

Chronic UI is the loss of urine that lasts more than 6 months and that is not definitively cured with the imposed treatment.

Urgent Urinary Incontinence (UUI)

In this way, UUI is called clinically with an urgent need to urinate. Although knowing the dynamic uro pattern is very important for therapeutics, today, the International Society for Incontinence has established the general name of overactive bladder, based on the clinic. The most frequent cause is the loss of the inhibition that the CNS exerts on the detrusor muscle. It is observed in cerebrovascular accidents, dementias, Parkinson's disease, etc. or in patients on benzodiazepines, antihistamines, and neuroleptics. Other causes of increased detrusor muscle contractions are local irritation of the bladder due to stones, cancer or infections and excessive distention of the bladder secondary to drugs (diuretics), or clinical situations (glucosuria) that increase urine volume. The UUI constitutes 50% to 75% of the causes of UI in women and men older than 75 years. The urgency to urinate is its characteristic symptom, and urinary losses can occur both day and night. In these patients, the postvoid residue after bladder emptying is small.

Stress Urinary Incontinence (SUI)

Stress incontinence is the product of a combination of factors that leads to greater laxity of the elements that make up the urogenital diaphragm (atrophy of the urethra epithelium and the trigone, sarcopenia) and herniation of the urethra. The latter acquires an extra-abdominal position, and its closure pressure is surpassed by bladder pressure during the Valsalva maneuver, which triggers the UI.

The anatomical changes secondary to multiparity and, in some cases, the presence of prolapses also predispose to deteriorate muscle tone in the pelvic floor. These factors lead to the development of greater laxity of the muscles that make up the urogenital diaphragm, which can facilitate the hypermobility of the urethra and the loss of the ability to achieve adequate continence in the face of increased intra-abdominal pressure. Normally, the urethra has an intra-abdominal location. This means that before certain maneuvers such as coughing or sneezing, there is an increase in intra-abdominal pressure that is transmitted simultaneously to the bladder and urethra. As both withstand the same pressure increase, urine does not leak. Now, when herniation of the urethra occurs, the pressure increase is transmitted only to the bladder (and not to the urethra, which is now in an extra-abdominal position). This pressure difference (higher in the bladder and lower in the urethra) makes the urine to easily escape. Patients who have bladder prolapse (cystocele) have the urethra located below the pelvic floor and, as a consequence, can present SUI, although the two situations can occur independently, or sometimes the prolapse conceals an underlying UI due to the distortion that produces in the anatomy of the urethra. The presence of atrophic vaginitis with irritation and bacterial colonization of the meatal area generates dysuria and worsens the symptoms of SUI. SUI is more frequent in women and constitutes the first cause of UI in women up to 75 years of age. After this age, the cause is mixed (SUI plus UUI). Characteristically, patients with SUI have incontinence when coughing, sneezing, laughing, or performing Valsalva maneuver and do not have losses during the night, when they are lying down. According to the degree of laxity, initially the losses occur at small efforts and in small volumes, but as the deterioration progresses, the losses are more noticeable. Since this type of incontinence does not alter the evacuation of urine, the postvoid residue measured by ultrasound is small.

Overflow Incontinence (OFI)

It occurs when intravesical pressure exceeds the mechanisms of sphincter restraint and can occur with or without bladder atony. In the first case, the contraction of the bladder is preserved, but there is an obstruction at the level of the urinary tract. In the second case, the bladder does not contract and the urine accumulates inside. As a consequence of any of these mechanisms, the large volume of urine accumulated inside the bladder generates pressure against the sphincter and ends up overflowing. The most common cause is benign prostatic hyperplasia (BPH), because the hypertrophied prostate reduces the urethral caliber and obstructs the bladder outlet tract. In these patients, the contraction of the bladder is initially preserved. It is important to note that although BPH is a prevalent entity, it is rare that it produces OFI. Other less frequent causes of OFI are diabetes mellitus or alcoholic neuropathy, cerebrovascular accidents, or spinal cord injuries that lead to OFI due to bladder atony. The history of pelvic surgery and pelvic radiotherapy should also be evaluated.

OFI occurs when the intravesical pressure exceeds the sphincteric containment mechanisms. This type of UI can occur without bladder atony (BPH) or with it (in diseases that affect the innervation of the detrusor, such as diabetes mellitus, stroke, or alcoholism).

OFI is the least prevalent cause of UI. It is more common in men older than 65 years, in whom it becomes the second cause of UI (after the urgent type). Patients with this type of UI have constant losses of small amounts of urine. At the beginning

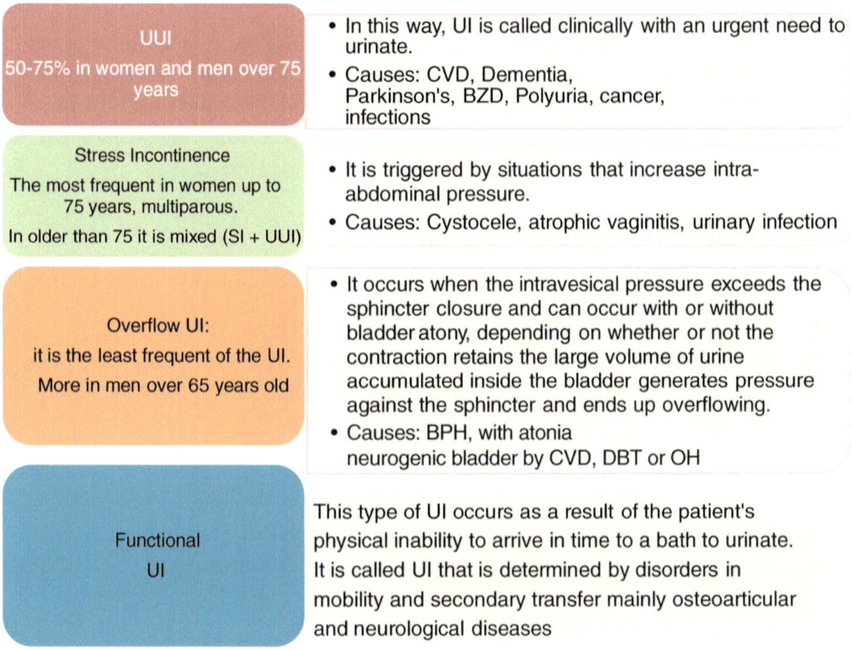

Fig. 6.4 Summary of the main types of permanent UI

they can refer pain or hypogastric discomfort. In these patients, the postvoid residue is increased. When the alteration is severe and does not resolve, it can lead to the development of hydronephrosis and subsequent obstructive renal failure (Fig. 6.4).

Functional Incontinence

This type of UI is produced as a consequence of the physical inability of the patient to arrive in time to a bath to urinate. It is determined by mobility and movement disorders secondary to stroke, Parkinson's disease, gait disorders, or social or family situations that make the patient to have no help to move or use appropriate devices when he/she wants to urinate. This type of UI depends on third parties to solve it.

Mixed Incontinence

It is one in which two types of UI are combined. It is very common to find women with UUI associated with SUI or men with UUI associated with OFI.

The prevalence of the different types of permanent UI varies according to the age and sex of the patients, although in general the causes are mixed. In women, it is more common to find SUI while in men, UUI and then OFI were more prevalent.

Evaluation of the Patient's Incontinence

- There is no formal recommendation to track UI in the older individuals; however, given the high prevalence and benefits of their treatment, several panels of experts recommend to ask patients over 65 about this problem, at least once.

Most causes of UI are diagnosed by asking and physical examination.

Interrogation

- The interrogation of the UI is technically simple, but it requires caution and care since it can happen that patients find it difficult to talk about this problem.
- It is fundamental to have an adequate doctor-patient relationship when facing the problem, to generate a consultation that guarantees the privacy of the older individual and to adopt a serious attitude when asking.
- It is also important to reassure the patient by clarifying that incontinence **is not a "normal" phenomenon of aging.**
- The UI is a multifactorial problem in the older individual, and the identification of potentially reversible or treatable situations can contribute to improve the management.
- The first goal in conducting the evaluation is to identify if the problem is transient or permanent, for it is necessary to ask in detail about the time of evolution of the UI and review (and detect or rule out) the causes of transient UI: irritation or inflammation around or in the lower urinary tract, increased urine output, medication effects, and situations that affect or impede the possibility or willingness to go to the bathroom.

It is recommended to use questions such as:

- *Do you have discomfort such as pain or burning when urinating?*
- *Do you urinate frequently and in small amounts?*

- *Is the amount of urine that you eliminate greater than what you routinely eliminated?*
- *Have you started using a new medication lately?*
- *Do you have difficulties accessing the bathroom at your home?*
- *Are you usually constipated?*

These questions allow the detection of transient UI causes such as urinary infections, polyuria, drugs, fecal bolus, etc. It is also advisable to carry out an exhaustive interrogation of the symptoms, the characteristics of the episodes, and the circumstances that produce or favor the UI, as well as to obtain a complete history of the drugs that the patient is taking at that moment. In the case of women, the number of pregnancies, the time of menopause, the history of pelvic surgeries, or local treatments with radiation should be noted. In men, it is essential to obtain prostatic and surgical records. In both cases, it should be recorded if there is a history of cognitive deterioration or previous confusional syndromes.

Through the interrogation, the doctor should try to define if the patient has transient or permanent UI and, in the case of the first one, what are the possible causes.

In patients with permanent UI, it will be necessary to define whether it is of urgency, effort, or overflow. There are certain types of questions whose response guides the doctor toward the cause of UI:

- *Do you lose urine when you cough, laugh, lift something, sneeze, or defecate?*
- *Do you wet your clothes or intimate towels, without realizing it, because you lose your urine?*
- *Can you stand 5 to 10 min until you reach a bathroom when you want to urinate?*
- *Do you lose urine when you go to the bathroom with extreme urgency?*
- *How often do you empty your bladder?*
- *How many times do you get up at night to urinate?* (You have to clarify if you wake up from the desire to urinate or if you have insomnia and then take advantage and go to the bathroom).
- *Do you feel that you empty your bladder completely every time you urinate?*
- *When you arrive at your house, when you open the entrance door, do you feel sudden urges to urinate, with occasional leakage of urine?* (key in lock syndrome).

If the patient has a sudden and urgent need to urinate, does not arrive in time to the bathroom, and has losses during the day and night, the most probable diagnosis is that of emergency UI. If the patient has a loss of urine when coughing, sneezing, laughing, or lifting and does not have losses during the night or when lying down, it is most likely a case of stressful UI. If the patient has constant losses of small amounts of urine and feels that it does not completely empty his bladder, he most likely has overflow incontinence.

Physical Exam

In the general evaluation, the ability of the older individual to move, use the bathroom, and deal with personal hygiene should be verified. In the functional evaluation, the patient should always be asked to evacuate his/her bladder beforehand and, if possible, record the volume urinated. To avoid confusion in the diagnosis of the type of UI, it is essential to make sure that the patient completely evacuated his/her bladder before examining it and, if there is doubt, proceed to determine the absence of residue. In the physical examination, the abdomen should be evaluated to verify the presence of diastasis of the anterior rectus muscles, which implies generalized muscular weakness, intra-abdominal masses, ascites, or any organomegaly, which increases the intra-abdominal pressure. The compression of the abdomen also serves to objectify the function of the lower urinary tract before the increase in pressure (an increase in intra-abdominal pressure is generated with a compressive maneuver of the hypogastrium, and it is seen if there are losses). A rectal examination should be included to identify the presence of a fecal bolus or alterations in anal sphincter tone and perineal sensitivity. In men, the morphology, size, and sensitivity of the prostate should be examined; in women, a gynecological examination should be included in search of pelvic masses, signs of atrophy of the vaginal mucosa, urogenital prolapse, or loss of the strength of the muscles of the urogenital diaphragm. Patients with atrophic vaginitis usually have a thin vaginal mucosa and, occasionally, petechiae. There may be vulvar atrophy, and the flow (if present) is aqueous or serosanguineous, with a pH greater than 4.5. The position of the urinary meatus should be evaluated at rest and during the Valsalva maneuver, to look for prolapse or UI when elevating the intra-abdominal pressure. A useful test to measure the strength of the muscles of the urogenital diaphragm is to ask the patient to contract the perineal muscles (she is told to try to contract the anal sphincter as when she wants to avoid gassing), and she is asked to keep the contraction for as long as possible. When the muscle strength is preserved, the woman can maintain the contraction for 5 to 10 seconds (making sure she does not use the accessory muscles that are the anterior rectus, the adductors, or the gluteal muscles). Neurological integrity should also be evaluated, particularly the anal tone (dependent on the nerve roots S4 and S5), the bulbocavernosus reflex (nerve roots S2 and S4), and the perineal sensitivity that depends on the same territory (S2 and S4).

In men, the bulbocavernosus reflex is taken by stimulating with a swab the skin near the middle raphe of the perineum, below the scrotal sac. In women, this reflex is taken in a gynecological position by applying the stimulus on the fold between the upper lip of the vagina and the thigh. In both cases, the normal response is the contraction of the anal sphincter before the stimulus. There is a very useful maneuver, which can be done in the office, which consists of asking the patient to come to the consultation with a full bladder (a previous 500 ml of water intake can be recommended) and examine it in a gynecological position. First you are asked to perform a Valsalva maneuver and observe if there is loss of urine through the urethral meatus and then the same is asked but lifting the urethra manually by touch and observing whether the loss continues or not. If loss is observed, a diagnosis of SUI is made; if it improves when the urethra is compressed, it suggests the possibility of a solution with devices or surgery. One strategy to sensitize the test is to ask the patient to perform the Valsalva maneuver, but when standing or in the position that the patient refers to us, incontinence occurs.

The physical examination of the patient is important since it serves to rule out the presence of bladder balloon, fecal bolus, or urogenital prolapse, determine the size and characteristics of the prostate, and review the gynecological and neurological integrity (whose alteration could cause UI).

Supplementary Exams

Among the complementary studies useful to evaluate patients with UI is the **urinalyses test and bladder ultrasound**. The analysis of urine allows physicians to detect the presence of glucosuria, hematuria, hypercalciuria, or signs of infection (pyuria). In cases in which the urinalysis suggests an infection, a urine culture should be obtained. Ultrasound is used to measure the postvoid residue. Characteristically, patients with SUI and UUI have a small postvoid residue, while in patients with OFI, the postvoid residue is high. However, it is not necessary to measure the postvoid residue in all patients, especially if the clinic is clear. In cases in which there are diagnostic doubts, the ultrasound is not easily accessible, and OFI is suspected (abdominal palpation reveals a bladder balloon whose compression arouses pain), the postvoid residue can be measured by placing a rigid sterile probe that will allow the evacuation of bladder contents and the objectification of their volume, since it should never rely on the simple physical examination in order to estimate the bladder residual volume.

The most useful tools to evaluate patients with UI are the interrogation and the physical examination, complemented with a urinalysis and, eventually, a bladder ultrasound when the clinic generates doubts.

In general, sophisticated tests, such as cystoscopy, imaging studies, or urodynamic tests, are usually not needed to evaluate the majority of outpatients, since these studies neither provide more complementary information nor lead to change the initiated therapy. In hospitalized patients, with more serious underlying diseases such as paraplegia, stroke sequelae, dementias, and postoperative gynecological or urological surgeries, these tests can help to achieve a correct interpretation of bladder function and its subsequent treatment.

Treatment of Urinary Incontinence

An adequate urine continence function and improved quality of life can be achieved, being this more important than the complete UI cure itself. UI is currently the geriatric syndrome with more therapeutic alterantives. UI therapeutic strategies can be divided into [20]:

- Behavioral measures
- Hygienic-dietetic measures
- Exercises for pelvic floor muscles
- Electrical stimulation
- Neuromodulation
- Intravaginal mechanical devices
- Pharmacological treatment potentially
- Surgical treatment

Behavioral Measures

The factors that are usually associated with the failure of bladder reeducation are the age and the severity of the UI, but the motivation and adherence to the interventions are crucial. The goals of bladder reeducation are to improve control over urgency, prolong the intervals between urinations, increase bladder capacity, reduce the number of episodes of UI, and restore the patient's confidence in the possibility of controlling bladder function. In ambulatory patients without cognitive impairment, the possibility of postponing micturition or adapting the micturition rhythm can be worked on, based on the urinary diary made by the patient. For this, the patient must begin to urinate, even without desire, at intervals less than the observed average; then it will increase by 15–30 min until an interval between urinations of approximately 3 h is reached. In institutionalized patients or patients with mild cognitive impairment, a fixed interval of urination can be established, and in cases of major deterioration or significant alterations in motility, the caregiver or nurse will take the patient to urinate at regular intervals. The basis of treatment should be behavioral work, since it has no undesirable effects, which are the main cause of discontinuation of pharmacological therapies.

Placebos

The role of placebo has been widely proven in the management of any UI type. In contrast to some concepts arising from classic studies, a recent study published in the Cochrane Library has established that the use of anticholinergics has been superior to the use of placebo to improve symptoms although, of course, it has more adverse effects.

Dietary Hygienic Measures

In the consultation, hygienic-dietetic measures aim to reduce the incontinence consequences. It is recomended to reduce drinks and foods rich in methylxanthines since they can promote urinary urgency, and to reduce alcohol intake since it is generally accepted that increases urine volume and, consequently, leads to higher urinary frequency, urgency, and finally incontinence. The water restriction from 18 to 19 hours helps to reduce the number of nocturnal voids in patients with nocturia. Proper hygienic protection is the first step against urine or fecal incontinence (the latter is the most frequently denied by patients). The Cochrane database has devoted a special chapter to the comparison between incontinence protectors.

Exercises for the Pelvic Floor Muscles (EPFM)

Rehabilitative treatment can be done through the Kegel exercises (*Arnold H. Kegel*), the electrical stimulation of the pelvic floor muscles, or mechanical devices. In ambulatory patients, the Kegel exercises and the placement of the mechanical devices can be taught, while the electrical stimulation is for more specialized centers. Kegel exercises are the most used physical therapy in the initial conservative treatment of SUI. These exercises increase the muscle tone of the pelvic muscles and achieves the urethra reposition. They are noninvasive, harmless, and inexpensive methods of treatment, although they may not be effective. In different studies, it was shown that they are as effective as electrical stimulation or estrogen therapy, and can even complement these therapies. They can be practiced in conjunction with any proposed treatment. The Cochrane Library performed systematic reviews including SUI, mixed urinary incontinence (MUI), and UUI, and the conclusion was that EPFMs are more effective than placebo or doing nothing. The benefits would not be superior with the addition of biofeedback, electrostimulation, vaginal cones, or anticholinergics; and young women, between 40 and 50 years of age, with SUI and participating in a supervised program for at least 3 months would be the most benefited, thus this strategy is considered to be the first line of treatment for this group.

How Are These Exercises Done?

First, the patient should be taught to correctly recognize diaphragmatic inspiration and expiration, because the contractions of the muscles should be performed during expiration. The increase in intra-abdominal pressure caused by the diaphragm in inspiration nullifies the strength of the pelvic muscle contraction with the least possible load on the part of the abdominal contents. Before starting, the patient should be relaxed, in position of abdominal discharge (lying down), for about 5 min. It is advisable to elevate the feet on a stool or similar with the knees bent at 90° and with a small pillow under the pelvis.

The patient should be taught to contract the muscles of the pelvic floor (obturator of the anus) in an active and voluntary way, without contracting other muscle groups (adductors, glutes, and abdominals mainly), because they have an antagonistic effect.

The exercises should be done in different positions, to adapt the patient to different conditions that can be found in their daily lives; the gravity effect must be worked from the supine standing position, taking its influence from zero to the maximum influence.

Intravaginal Mechanical Devices

Exercising the pelvic floor muscles can be done alone or with the help of devices. In addition to the perineometry machines with or without biofeedback devices, there are vaginal cones or any other type of intravaginal devices, which consist of placing cones of different weight in the vagina, the purpose of which is to be retained in place by the EMPP or some device to be "tightened" by the contraction of the muscles. The Cochrane Library established that, although they are useful, they are not superior to the EMPP alone, especially considering their high abandonment rate.

Electrical Stimulation

The electrical stimulation consists in the application of brief stimuli by means of small needles or surface electrodes. They are useful in urge incontinence and effort incontinence. In some countries, it is considered as an alternative for those cases in which a properly performed EPFM has failed. However, the Cochrane study of 2003 did not show benefits with the addition of electrostimulation to the EPFM.

Neuromodulation

The neuromodulation of the sacral nerve is a valuable treatment for those patients who suffer from urge incontinence refractory to all types of treatment, but its high cost, for the moment, makes it an almost inaccessible alternative to most patients.

Anti-incontinence Devices

Anti-incontinence devices were developed for the treatment of SUI, but they are also useful in women with symptoms of urgency. The most developed are the intra-vaginal pessaries. The pessaries consist of silicone rings that are attached to a "knob," in order to generate some type of obstruction either fixed or dynamic in the posterior wall of the urethra. The optimal size, which ensures both continence and adequate bladder emptying, is chosen by performing UI tests with the bladder filled with the pessary placed [17].

Pharmacological Treatment of Urinary Incontinence

Drug therapy for the treatment of UI is widely used for urge incontinence and mixed incontinence if behavioral therapy is not effective. Few agents are available for stress incontinence. The drugs used can be divided into two large groups: hormones and drugs designed to increase the storage capacity of urine, by either detrusor relaxation, increased intraurethral pressure, or both. Incontinence of transitory urine, usually caused by urinary infections or other causes of simple intervention, should always be considered.

Management of Acute Incontinence

The treatment of acute incontinence depends on its cause. Within the assessment of the causes of acute UI, a functional assessment of the patient should be made to determine mobility, transfer capacity, manual dexterity, and correct hygiene capacity. On the other hand, the presence of depression should also be investigated and the cognitive status determined for proper planning of problem management.

General Support Measures

If a fecal bolus is detected, it is indicated to evacuate it. If UI is due to the use of drugs, it is advisable to reevaluate the indication of the drug or reduce the dose; in cases of polyuria, the underlying disease should be treated. Those patients who have UI in the context of depressive or behavioral symptoms require an interdisciplinary approach. The treatment of the underlying disease will resolve the UI, then no specific treatment is required for the urinary tract.

Urinary Infections

Urinary infection is very prevalent in women. It is estimated that around 15% to 20% of postmenopausal women will have a urinary tract infection sometimes after that. The prevalence of asymptomatic bacteriuria also increases with age. Thus, at 40 years, their estimated rate is around 5%, a figure that contrasts with an average 50% in women aged 75 or older. Taking these data into account is crucial, since in this group of women, and in the absence of overt urological disease, the bacteriuria should not be treated since its chance of recurrence is close to 100%, especially when it comes to the presence of *Escherichia coli*. The treatment is not very different from that of younger patients, and the drugs used are trimethoprim-sulfamethoxazole (TMS) or nitrofurantoin, if they are not contraindicated (e.g., allergy). With the short schemes (3 days), the same effectiveness is usually achieved (cure and relapse rate), greater adherence, lower costs, and less incidence of adverse effects than with conventional treatments of 5 to 7 days. Adverse effects are rare when the 3-day treatment schedule is used. The dose should be reduced in renal failure.

The TMS is the drug of choice for the treatment of uncomplicated urinary tract infections in ambulatory older patients and with no history of urogenital diseases (if it is not contraindicated). This treatment is effective, easily adherent, and usually well tolerated.

A therapeutic scheme based on nitrofurantoin is the most cumbersome since it requires four daily doses that can compromise adherence to treatment. It is contraindicated in patients with creatinine clearance less than 40 ml/min. Quinolones are second-line drugs in the treatment of low urinary tract infections in the ambulatory older patient and are first line when there is resistance to TMS greater than 20% in the medium being treated. Norfloxacin can be used orally for 3 days. It is usually well tolerated but can cause nausea, vomiting, abdominal discomfort, headache, and skin rash. Ciprofloxacina is used in male patients and for a period of 7 days, especially if they carry BPH. Of course, the above mentioned antibiotics can be used if they are not contraindicated.

Quinolones should be used when the drugs of first choice are ineffective or produce intolerance or the patient has a history of allergy to them.

Management of Chronic Urinary Incontinence

Urgent Urinary Incontinence

Hormone Treatment

The role of hormone replacement treatment for UI is controversial. The treatment of urogenital atrophy can be carried out in a safe, simple way and looking for the lowest possible dose. Its objective is to improve tissue trophism and reduce symptoms such as vaginal dryness, burning, and itching, all of which improve the quality of life of the woman, and, secondarily, both the symptoms of urgency, frequency, or those attributable to the recurrent urinary tract infection present a gradual improvement. In general terms it is preferable to use local estrogens over general ones (Table 6.5). This allows the use of low doses of estrogen replacement hormones, with a high degree of local action, without promoting endometrial proliferation and avoiding the need to use protection with progestogens, whose effect on the urinary tree is controversial. The maximum effect is reached around 12 weeks of application. Once the desired effect is obtained, a maintenance dose is left in order not to lose the benefits achieved.

The Cochrane systematic review updated in 2005 concluded that the use of estrogens can improve or even can cure incontinence, although evidence suggests that this effect is mainly attributable to urge urinary incontinence. The combination of estrogen with progesterone would not seem to improve UI but would actually reduce cure rates and improvement. Estrogen therapy, especially local, improves urgency, day and night frequency, and episodes of incontinence in patients with symptoms suggestive of overactive bladder. Treatment consists of a daily application for 2 or 3 weeks at least, although sometimes intensive treatment should be longer to achieve remission of symptoms. If the symptoms remit, the patient will continue with the maintenance administration (usually 1 or 2 weekly applications). Adverse effects of local hormonal treatment are exceptional and include local irritation, secondary candidiasis, and, less frequently, bleeding or breast tenderness [6, 7, 10, 11, 14–19].

Table 6.5 Estrogens available for local treatment

Presentation	Drug
Ovules	Estriol
	Promestriene
Creams	Estriol
	Promestriene
	Conjugated equine estrogens

Nonhormonal Treatment

The main objective of pharmacological treatment is to treat UUI, although in the last few years some drugs have been developed to treat stress incontinence. The treatment of UUI is special, since the bladder filling volume that triggers incontinence is characteristic of each patient. The goal is to define that threshold and tell the patient to evacuate the bladder before overcoming it. A pharmacological treatment should also be indicated in order to reduce muscle contractions, either by acting directly on the bladder muscle or by increasing the inhibitory effect at the level of the CNS. Anticholinergics are, so far, the most used and effective for the urgent UI treatment, which makes them the first choice for the overactive bladder treatment. They have been shown to be effective in reducing symptomatology in numerous randomized trials in which they were compared with placebos. Its effectiveness lies in inhibiting the involuntary contractions of the detrusor by antagonizing the muscarinic receptors of the parasympathetic pathway. Anticholinergics should be handled with caution in patients with dementia and in those women who receive psychotropic drugs, because of their potential adverse effects. They are also contraindicated in patients with narrow-angle glaucoma and in cases of obstruction of the urinary tract. The most active drug and considered the standard one is *oxybutynin*, a nonselective anticholinergic available in oral presentations (immediate-release or prolonged-release formulations), transdermal patches and transvaginal, transrectal and intravesical applications. Oxybutynin is poorly tolerated by the older patients because of its anticholinergic effects such as sedation and weakness. Effectiveness in doses adequately tolerated by the older individuals is questioned (except in the extended-release formulations). This drug is classified by BEERS criteria inappropriate for use in geriatric patients (high risk of severity). Regarding *tolterodine*, it has greater selectivity for bladder cholinergic receptors and, therefore, fewer systemic effects such as constipation and mouth dryness, also available in oral presentation of immediate-release or prolonged-release formulations. In a systematic review published in the Cochrane Library, which analyzed studies of high methodological quality that compared oxybutynin with tolterodine, both in their presentation of immediate release, no significant difference was found between them in terms of efficacy, close to 60%. However, fewer side effects such as dry mouth were described with tolterodine. The prolonged-release presentations have a lower adverse effect rate than the classical ones, so if available, they should be preferred. With respect to other anticholinergics, the different studies provide little data to establish a conclusion. Both drugs can produce cognitive impairment, although it would be less with tolterodine. Regarding *trospium chloride,* in multicenter studies, it has been shown that the efficacy of this anticholinergic agent is similar to that of oxybutynin with immediate effect. The rate of abandonment due to undesirable effects, mainly dry mouth, is slightly lower than that of other anticholinergics.

Solifenacin is the anticholinergic with greater selectivity for M3 receptors of the bladder. Studies have shown that it is well tolerated, and it has an immediate effect, slightly higher rate of reduction in urgency symptoms and frequency, as well as in episodes of incontinence, compared to tolterodine. Its metabolism occurs in the liver and has interactions with drugs such as ketoconazole, which is often used in incontinent patients. So far it has shown no effect on the CNS similar to other anticholinergics. *Darifenacin* is a drug with high selectivity for M3 receptors by acting as selective antagonist of M3 subtype muscarinic receptors limiting bladder contractions, reducing symptoms of hyperactivity and vesical irritability as urge incontinence, frequency and urgency, with little effect on the salivary glands and almost no effect on the CNS and cardiovascular system. These characteristics would make it an attractive drug to be used in older individuals due to its few undesirable effects and the possibility of being used in patients with cognitive impairment medicated with psychotropic drugs. However, it shares hepatic metabolism with antidepressants, so it should be handled with caution in patients who receive them. It was approved by FDA for the treatment of overactive bladder in December 2004. The preliminary results attribute an effectiveness comparable to tolterodine with immediate effect, with very good tolerance and low dropout rate due to adverse effects. Given the hepatic metabolism that the drug has, its dose should be reduced in patients with hepatic impairment Child-Pugh B, and its use is not recommended in hepatic patients Child-Pugh C. In a randomized study of 445 patients, the average number of episodes of urge incontinence per week decreased more with darifenacin than with placebo. In a subanalysis of a data pool of phase III studies with varying doses of darifenacin, an efficacy superior to placebo was found in the reduction of incontinence in geriatric patients. Several adverse effects on the CNS have been reported, such as headache, confusion, hallucinations, and drowsiness, related to the use of darifenacin. These effects were observed particularly at the beginning of the treatment and/or when increasing the dose.

The Argentine National Pharmacovigilance System has not received reports of any of the adverse effects related to darifenacin above indicated. This administration recommends:

- Warn patients, especially if they are older, that they should not drive vehicles or use heavy machinery, until they know if darifenacin produces effects on the CNS.
- Suspend the treatment or consult the attending physician if adverse reactions such as confusion, hallucinations, and/or drowsiness occur.

This alert does not invalidate its use but makes it more specific, and these patients should be more controlled, especially since the dropout rate due to adverse effects with this drug is low. Darifenacin is the drug that showed a more adequate ratio for the selectivity of muscarinic receptors of the bladder compared with those of salivary glands (M3 vs. M1) [8–12].

Local Suppressors of Bladder Smooth Muscle

Within this group are tricyclic antidepressants, particularly *imipramine*, which reduces bladder contractility and increases output resistance. Its mechanism of action would be the direct suppression of bladder muscle activity. As these drugs have a narrow margin of safety, with significant adverse effects, they should be handled with great caution in older patients, especially due to its cardiovascular toxicity.

Central Action Drugs

Within the multiple sites of action of the *5-hydroxytryptamine* (*serotonin*), are the motor cells of the lumbosacral medulla, where they exert a stimulating effect on sympathetic nerves and an inhibitory effect on parasympathetic nerves, increasing the bladder capacity and favor continence. Several inhibitors of serotonin reuptake are under investigation, however *fluoxetine* and *venlafaxine* have been investigated, finding that they have no beneficial effect on UI, conversely favoring incontinence by alpha-blocking effect [4].

Drugs of Intravesical Action

Oxybutynin bladder instillations are effective for the treatment of overactive bladder in patients with poor response to oral treatment or poor tolerance to the drug. This route of administration would have a high rate of effectiveness, with fewer adverse effects due to its low systemic absorption and low levels of circulating metabolites due to lack of the first hepatic step. Despite all these, there are no randomized controlled trials that demonstrate these benefits; also, the need to catheterize three to four times a day makes this route of administration poorly accepted and with low adherence to treatment. The use of local anesthetics such as *lidocaine* to decrease bladder activity is highly effective, but with very short duration effects, which is why it is not useful for long-term treatments. The *botulinum toxin* naturally produced by Gram-positive anaerobic bacillus *Clostridium botulinum* has been used since 1980 in various therapeutic applications. The toxins commercialized for urological use available in the market are type A and type B. For the treatment of overactive bladder, the injectable form is used through fibrocystoscopy, applying it at 30 different detrusor sites, avoiding the bladder trigone area. In general, the used doses are low, and the duration of the effect as well as the undesirable effects are dose-dependent. The chemical denervation generated is not permanent, since between 6 and 16 weeks it usually produces a reinnervation from collateral axons. The studies available to date show that botulinum toxin is an effective option for the treatment of neurogenic and non-neurogenic overactive bladder in those patients who do not respond to the use of anticholinergics. The benefit of its application in the urethral sphincter for the treatment of vesicourethral dyssynergia has also been demonstrated. The use of botulinum toxin is not approved so far in diseases of the lower urinary tract, although the publications suggest its usefulness. Even more randomized trials with adequate methodological quality are needed to validate its application and evaluate adverse effects. Generally, UUI treatment is lifelong and its objective is that the patient does not have any accidental urine leakage, and in very old patients or patients severely compromised in their general health by other diseases, a reasonable goal is that the daily losses are reduced as much as possible, and that the patients accomplishe a comfortable sleep [13].

Stress Urine Incontinence (SUI) Treatment

The initial treatment of SUI is based on fortifying the pelvic musculature using Kegel perineal exercises. These simple exercises consist in making regular contractions of the perineal floor musculature. Patients who perform Kegel exercises regularly for 15 to 21 days achieve up to 70% improvement in symptoms, and this can be maintained if the patient continues exercising daily. Kegel exercises are also effective for patients with mild urogenital prolapse.

> Kegel exercises are an excellent therapeutic option for patients with mild SUI without urogenital prolapse or with mild prolapse.

One option for patients who cannot perform the exercises is to offer them a rehabilitation therapy by electrical stimulation of the perineal muscles through an intravaginal or intra-anal device. This method has an efficacy similar to Kegel exercises but requires trained personnel and the disposition of the patient. Another therapeutic option is local estrogens, since systemic administration is currently contraindicated, improving urethral trophism and reducing SUI. They also increase the population of receptors α 1 periurethral (this would allow effective use of α-stimulating drugs) [5].

Drugs for Stress Urinary Incontinence

Several drugs have been evaluated, and among the most prominent is the adrenergic group, such as *ephedrine*, *pseudoephedrine*, and *phenylpropanolamine,* which promote continence by favoring contraction of the smooth muscle of the urethra and the bladder neck, increasing the pressure of urethral closure. The Cochrane Library conducted a systematic review of the topic, concluding that the evidence available to date is weak enough to suggest that the treatment is superior to placebo. The *duloxetine* is approved for use as an antidepressant and is under review by the FDA for incontinence treatment.

It inhibits the reuptake of serotonin and noradrenaline, increasing its concentration in the spinal cord and amplifying the activity of the pudendal nerve. Randomized studies with a larger number of patients show a reduction in incontinence episodes between 54% and 64% versus 41% in the placebo group. Duloxetine also has very good results in post-prostatectomy urinary incontinence [4–9].

The treatment of choice for SUI patients without urogenital prolapse or with small prolapse is Kegel exercises, eventually associated with local estrogens. In patients with grade III and IV prolapse, the specialist should be consulted to define the resolution of the problem. The definitive resolution is always surgical.

Urine Incontinence Due to Overflow (OFI)

The treatment of OFI depends on the cause that originates it; if it is obstructive, secondary to prostatic hypertrophy, the initial treatment can be with drugs or with desobstructive surgery; the recommendation should be given taking into account the patient's preferences after explaining the advantages and disadvantages of the therapeutic procedures. Two types of drugs are available for OFI treatment: α-adrenergic blockers and finasteride. The administration of finasteride, in a single daily dose, reduces obstructive symptoms, increases urinary flow, and decreases prostate size by 25% after 3 to 6 months of treatment. Finasteride is useful only in patients with large prostates (size greater than 40 cc) and, if used for several years, decreases the risk of acute urinary retention and need of surgery. If pharmacological treatment was the first choice and it fails, the urologist should be consulted to seek surgical resolution of the problem.

Obstructive OFI can be treated pharmacologically (with α-adrenergic blockers or finasteride) or by surgery. The choice of treatment will depend on the patients' desire and their functional status and comorbidities.

When the OFI is nonobstructive, that is to say that it is produced by bladder atony, a pharmacological treatment can be tried or, alternatively, opt for the instrumental evacuation of the bladder. In older patients, the latter option is preferred since pharmacological treatments have many cardio-stimulant effects and can produce tachycardia, hypertension, and arrhythmias, which is why they are currently in disuse.

Functional Urinary Incontinence (FUI)

In functional urinary incontinence, the problem solution is outside the urinary tract, as it is resolved by taking measures which facilitate patient access to the bathroom, bringing a potty closer, training their caregivers, implementing building reforms that improve their movement, place comfortable clothes, education, training of caregivers etc.

Conclusion

Urinary incontinence is considered one of the most frequent chronic problems in outpatients with maximum expression in the older individuals. Among its pathophysiology and classification, the most important thing still is "think about it and make the correct question." UI is one of that called Giants of Geriatrics (Inmobility, Instability, Intellectual impairment and Incontinence), described by Bernard Isaccs in the seventies, in UK.

References

1. Tobin GW. Incontinence in the elderly. 1st ed. Londres, Reino Unido: Edward Arnold; 1995.
2. Hunskaar S, Lose G, et al. Prevalence of Stress Urinary Incontinence in Women in Four European Countries, 2002. ICS: UK. 2003. Link to PDF: http://www.icsoffice.org/publications/2002/pdf/257.pdf (Acceso 28.11.2006).
3. Denis L, et al. Continence promotion: prevention, education and organisation. In Abrams P, et al (eds) Third International Consultation on Incontinence, Monaco. 2004; vol 1, p. 43.
4. Alhasso A y col. Adrenergic drugs for urinary incontinence in adults. Cochrane Database Syst Rev. 2005;(2):CD001842.
5. Burgio K y col. Behavioral training with and without biofeedback in the treatment of urge incontinence in older women: a randomized controlled trial. JAMA. 2002;288:2293–9.
6. Cardozo L y col. A systematic review of the effects of estrogens for symptoms suggestive of overactive bladder. Acta Obstet Gynecol Scand. 2004;83:892–7.
7. Cardozo L y col. Meta-analysis of estrogen therapy in the management of urogenital atrophy in postmenopausal women: second report of the Hormones and Urogenital Therapy Committee. Obstet Gynecol. 1998;92(4 Pt 2):722–7.
8. Diokno A y col. Prospective, randomized, double-blind study of the efficacy and tolerability of the extended-release formulations of oxybutynin and tolterodine for overactive bladder: results of the OPERA trial. Mayo Clin Proc. 2003;78:687–95.
9. Dmochowski R y col. Duloxetine versus placebo for the treatment of North American women with stress urinary incontinence. J Urol. 2003;170:1259–63.
10. Fantl J y col. Estrogen therapy in the management of urinary incontinence in postmenopausal women: a meta-analysis. First report of the Hormones and Urogenital Therapy Committee. Obstet Gynecol. 1994;83:12–8.
11. Grady D y col. Postmenopausal hormones and incontinence, The heart and/Progestin Replacement Study. Obstet Gynecol. 2001;97:116–20.
12. Hay-Smith J y col. Which anticholinergic drug for overactive bladder symptoms in adults. Cochrane Database Syst Rev. 2005;(3):CD005429.
13. Leippold T y col. Botulinum toxin as new therapy option for voiding disorders: current state of the art. Eur Urol. 2003;44:165–74.
14. Moehrer B y col. Oestrogens for urinary incontinence in women. Cochrane Database Syst Rev. 2003;(2):CD001405.
15. Molander y col. An epidemiological study of urinary incontinence and related urogenital symptoms in elderly women. Maturitas. 1990;12:51–60.
16. North American Menopause Society. Amended report from the NAMS advisory panel on postmenopausal hormone therapy. Menopause. 2003;10(1):6–12.
17. Pott-Grinstein E y col. Gynecologists' patterns of prescribing pessaries. J Reprod Med. 2001;46(3):205–8.

18. Speroff L y col. Practical guidelines for postmenopausal hormone therapy. Maturitas. 2005;51:4–7.
19. Suckling J y col. Local oestrogen for vaginal atrophy in postmenopausal women. Cochrane Database Syst Rev. 2006;(4):CD001500.
20. Tam H y col. Newer pharmacologic options in management of overactive bladder syndrome. Curr Opin Obstet Gynecol. 2005;17:495–506.

Chapter 7
Polypharmacy and the Older Patient: The Clinical Pharmacologist Perspective

Paula Scibona, Maria Valeria Beruto, Nadia E. Savoy, and Ventura A. Simonovich

Introduction

Advances in medical technology, new surgical procedures, and clinical practices as well as the development of new drugs and therapies have increased expectancy and quality of life of the general population, so, in recent decades, there has been a significant increase in older patients.

This leads to an increase in the prevalence of chronic diseases and greater requirement for simultaneous therapeutic strategies. Therefore, doctors are more often challenged to face these situations in which chronic diseases are overlap, such as cardiovascular disorders, arthritis, diabetes mellitus, dementia, hypertension and cancers, among others, making polypharmacy something possibly necessary.

Different drug schemes are widely used in all age groups, but pharmacokinetic and pharmacodynamic changes related to age and the high rate of comorbidities that these concomitant pharmacological interventions require put older people at greater risk of drug interactions, adverse effects, and inadequate doses. It is also associated with a higher probability of hospitalization and morbimortality such as falls, fractures, bleeding, and delirium [1].

Polypharmacy

There is no global consensus on the specific definition of polypharmacy, although different definitions have been adopted in different bibliographic reviews.

P. Scibona (✉) · M. V. Beruto · N. E. Savoy · V. A. Simonovich
Clinical Pharmacology Section, Hospital Italiano de Buenos Aires, Buenos Aires, Argentina
e-mail: paula.scibona@hospitalitaliano.org.ar

© Springer Nature Switzerland AG 2021

C. G. Musso et al. (eds.), *Frailty and Kidney Disease*,
https://doi.org/10.1007/978-3-030-53529-2_7

The World Health Organization (WHO) defines polypharmacy as the simultaneous administration of *several* medications to the same patient [2], although the exact number of medications used to define "polypharmacy" is variable and not determined.

In general, polypharmacy tends to be considered in quantitative terms, but we believe it is important to consider the qualitative aspects of it as well. A King's Fund report attempts to classify polypharmacy as appropriate or problematic. It defines as appropriate the prescription for complex or multiple conditions, in which the use of medications has been optimized and the medications are prescribed according to the best evidence, that is, with the intention of improving the quality of life and longevity and minimizing the damage. On the other hand, the same report defines problematic polypharmacy as the inappropriate prescription of multiple medications, or the non-obtaining of the expected benefit of the medication, through non-evidence-based therapy, unfavorable risk-benefit balance, dangerous interactions, unacceptable treatment, or poor adherence, among other causes [3].

In the course of this chapter, we will consider polypharmacy as the prescription of five or more drugs at any time, as a quantitative distinction [4], and/or that any of these is used without clinical justification, as a qualitative distinction [5].

Epidemiology of Polypharmacy

Polypharmacy is an increasing condition along all stages of life as seen in high- and medium-income countries, with estimates that show a prevalence between 40% and 50% in older adults [6]. There are a number of factors that are still under study in terms of their role in polypharmacy, such as nursing home admission, in which the evidence is contradictory whether it increases or not the risk of polypharmacy. Other factors, such as number of prescribers and frailty, are definitely associated with a higher risk of polypharmacy. Some studies have found that the number of medications increases between 60 and 80 years old and starts to decline after the age of 85 years old, which depicts an inverted U-shaped association between age and number of drugs [7].

There are still many gaps of knowledge in terms of the epidemiology of polypharmacy not only because we lack prospective studies designed to specifically measure incident and prevalent polypharmacy but also because it is very difficult to determine the impact of polypharmacy in an aging cohort with multiple comorbidities. In this sense, confounders are one of the many biases that may challenge these types of studies.

However, with a conservative perspective, it is estimated that drug-drug interactions occur in 13% of patients with polypharmacy. When the number of drugs raises to ten or more, the chance to have a potentially serious interaction climbs to 30% [8]. Consequently, the number of adverse drug reactions increases not only for the effect of the individual drugs but also for the interactions between them. One of the main drivers for adverse drug reactions and for unplanned hospitalization is polypharmacy.

When assessing polypharmacy, it is of great importance to evaluate the use of nonprescription medications in older adults, as well as herbal remedies and nutritional supplements. Older adults should be warned about the possibility of experiencing drug-drug interactions and adverse drug reactions between their prescribed medications and any other non-prescribed, herbal, or nutritional formula. On the other hand, physicians should be encouraged to identify unnecessary drug use and deprescribe. Several studies show that there is a high prevalence of patients that have suboptimal or lack of indication for drugs that they are consuming. There are also patients that have been prescribed with ineffective drugs for their conditions or therapeutic duplication in their medication regimens. This can be assessed by the Medication Appropriateness Index (MAI) criteria. The reasons for the unnecessary drug use included no indication (32%), lack of effectiveness (18%), and therapeutic duplication (7%). Gastrointestinal, central nervous system, and therapeutic nutrient/mineral agents were found to be the most commonly used unnecessary drugs [9]. Even worse, another study showed that there is a high prevalence of medication underuse, meaning that some patients are not receiving medications for which they have a clear indication, and that some of these patients experience unnecessary use as well. In other words, there are patients, around 40% of the patients with polypharmacy, that are prescribed with unnecessary drugs and not prescribed with drugs that they really need.

In Sweden, a 2012 study identified the 20 most commonly prescribed medications in the general population of people aged ≥65 years and revealed that these medications were used by up to 35% of older adults. Several of these medications were associated with falls, including hypnotics, sedatives, antidepressants, opioids, and other nonsteroidal analgesics and anti-inflammatories, antipsychotics, thiazide diuretics, angiotensin-converting enzyme (ACE) inhibitors, thyroid hormones, and medications for constipation [10].

In 2012, a Canadian study concludes that medications that increase the risk of falls include medications for cardiovascular diseases (e.g., digoxin, antiarrhythmics, and type 1a diuretics), benzodiazepines, antidepressants, antiepileptics, antipsychotics, antiparkinsonians, opioids, and urological spasmolytics. These drugs have a wide spectrum of adverse effects, so it should take particular care and prioritize the need for treatment [11].

Scores to Assess Polypharmacy

There are different tools for assessing inappropriate prescribing, the majority focusing on the older population, that is, Beers' criteria, STOPP (Screening Tool of Older People's potentially inappropriate Prescriptions), START (Screening Tool to Alert doctors to Right Treatment), Medication Appropriateness Index, comorbidity-polypharmacy score (CPS), or a combination. None of these tools are specifically designed to assess the liability of polypharmacy although some are arguably better suited to this. Importantly, it is useless to measure polypharmacy if comorbidities are not measured in view that we face the emergence of a twin phenomenon: multi-morbidity and polypharmacy. Comorbidities may be included at the polypharmacy score, as in the CPS, or may be measured by specific scores, as Charlson's score. However, there is room for improvement in the development of tools to measure not only the quantity and appropriateness of prescribed drugs but also the risk associated with the prescription [12].

Pharmacological Considerations with Impact on Polypharmacy

Pharmacokinetics and Dynamics

Pharmacokinetics studies the processes carried out by drugs within the body from the moment they enter until they are eliminated; these processes are absorption, distribution, metabolism, and elimination.

Pharmacodynamics studies the actions and effects of different drugs in the body and its mechanism of action.

Even in the absence of a specific disease, the passage of time is associated with different changes in both kinetics and pharmacodynamics, which may predispose to variations in the response to drugs, increasing the incidence of adverse effects [13].

Around the age of 40, changes in body composition begin: muscle mass decreases, fat increases, liver function alters, decrease in renal function progressively begins, and there is a progressive reduction in total body water, gastrointestinal motility reduction, and blood flow and gastric acid secretion. All these changes are accentuated as people get older and can affect the kinetics of drugs. However, the net effect of all these changes is difficult to predict [14].

Intestinal changes such as decreased motility, flow, and acid secretion can affect the absorption of different drugs, especially those that depend on an acidic medium to be absorbed.

Changes related to total body water and fat can affect the distribution of drugs. The decrease in total body water generates a decrease in the volume of distribution (Vd) for hydrophilic drugs, while the increase in total body fat produces a 20–40% increase in Vd for lipophilic drugs [15, 16].

On the other hand, it is known that the volume of distribution (Vd) increases with age, partly due to a decrease in protein-binding and mainly due to a relative increase in fat [17]. However, the increase in the free plasma fraction and the decrease in total clearance compensate the effect of aging on Vd [18].

The vast majority of drugs present before being eliminated some type of metabolism, mainly at the liver level and particularly by the microsomal system. Changes in liver volume and blood flow determine a reduction in metabolic reactions, particularly those known collectively as Phase I, catalyzed by cytochrome P450 enzymes (CYP450), which in turn can reduce total and drug-free elimination [19–21].

At the same time, liver metabolism is where drug interactions occur most frequently.

The main route of drug elimination is renal, which, in turn, is the most sensitive to age-related physiological changes and is also a route subject to potential interactions.

Physiologically there is a progressive reduction in the glomerular filtration rate (GFR). The reduction of glomerular filtration rate (GFR) secondary to aging begins around 30 years and continues to decrease at a rate of approximately 1 mL/year. It should be noted that this reduction in GFR is not reflected in serum creatinine and urea levels; they usually have normal values [22]. Similarly, the effective renal plasma flow (ERPF) is reduced in the course of life, reaching up to 50% in older people.

This progressive decrease in GFR is associated with a prolongation of the half-life (T1/2) of different non-lipophilic drugs that have a predominantly renal clearance [22, 23]. The measurement or estimation of creatinine clearance or GFR should always be done before starting any new drug to perform dose adjustment. Reduction of renal clearance of drugs may result in an increased risk of dose-dependent adverse effects [24, 25].

On the other hand, over the years, the capacity of secretion of the tubules is reduced; this must be taken into account for those medications that are excreted by renal secretion to avoid the accumulation of these drugs [26].

Because the physiological changes have an impact on the kinetics of most of the prescribed drugs, they must always be kept in mind when indicating, assessing adverse reactions and eventual dangerous interactions.

According to the aforementioned changes, there are different strategies to consider at the time of prescription: reduction of individual doses, increase in the inter-dose interval, or a combination of both, depending on whether the area under the curve (AUC) or maximum concentration (Cmax) is the main pharmacokinetic characteristics associated with efficacy and/or toxicity [27].

Pharmacodynamics

Pharmacodynamics may also change over time, mainly in relation to drug sensitivity. The same pharmacokinetic concentration in the biophase may produce reduced or, more frequently, increased effects (usually adverse effects) in older patients compared to younger patients [24]. This, in turn, may suggest the need for further dose reductions for some medications. In contrast, in some cases, older patients show less sensitivity, for instance, with medications that affect beta-adrenergic receptors. Except for antimicrobials, the preferred therapeutic approach in older patients has generally been to "start low and go slow" to avoid adverse effects. However, this poses risks for a possible suboptimal therapy [25, 28].

Pharmacogenetics and Therapeutic Drug Monitoring (TDM)

The pharmacological effects depend on the result of a series of pharmacokinetic processes, which determine how much drug reaches the biophase (target tissues), and pharmacodynamics, which involves the interaction between drug and its site of action [26]. These processes occur at a variable rate in different individuals and depend on many factors including sex, age, diet, environmental factors, pharmacological interactions, demography, and clinic, but one of the main determinants of this variability is the genetic. The structure, function, and expression of most of the enzymes involved in the transport and metabolism of the medications, as well as the specific receptors of the medications, can be affected by the presence of genetic variants, which in turn can modify the effect of planned therapeutic or the occurrence of adverse effects [29].

Genetic factors contribute to response variability in various ways, since they encode proteins involved in drug transport and their metabolism, or in the specific receptors on which the different drugs act. The genetic variants could have an impact on the therapeutic response to different drugs, which are mainly those of the cytochrome P450 superfamily. This superfamily is composed of a set of enzymes that perform reactions of oxidoreduction in the metabolism and are involved in the elimination of endogenous compounds and various drugs. The genes that encode these enzymes may have variants in the sequence that condition the response to the different drugs.

The biotransformation of drugs in the older population is more likely to be the basis of an adverse reaction when the family of liver enzymes P450 is involved. It is known that many medications are inducers or inhibitors of this enzyme system. Therefore, in theory, even with a drug that a patient has tolerated well, there is the possibility of an adverse reaction when a second drug is added that also intervenes in this metabolic pathway.

The research of these genetic variants prior to drug administration would help predict the patient's response. This concept represents the central objective of pharmacogenomics. However, pharmacogenetic knowledge does not explain all the variability in responses to medications [29]. Consequently, therapy must combine genetic information and non-genetic factors.

TDM refers to the individualization of the dosage of drugs within a therapeutic range and involves the measurement of plasma or serum drug concentrations. TDM is very useful since patients can respond differently to the same dosage regimen, depending on the changes and variability in the absorption, distribution, and elimination of the drug, such as the pediatric population, critical patients, and older individuals.

The aging process implies a progressive loss of the functional capacities of the organs, and this leads to changes in kinetics [30, 31]. In addition, older patients have a greater susceptibility to the toxic effects of medications. The unexpected or altered response to medications in this group compared to younger individuals can be mainly explained by changes in pharmacokinetics, dynamic changes, or pharmacological interactions [30]. In turn, there are many different clinical scenarios (sepsis, cardiac arrhythmias, etc.) in older patients which can further modify these processes so that they could benefit from therapeutic drug monitoring [29].

Polypharmacy-Related Risks

The risk of occurrence of adverse drug events increases with each new drug added to the treatment regimen, and, the greater the number of medications consumed, the greater the risk of occurrence of a clinically severe drug interaction [21]. As we already commented, older adults frequently receive a large number of medications prescribed by one or more professionals, beyond that of unnecessary costs, polypharmacy puts this population at risk of dangerous drug interactions and greater adverse effects.

Adverse effects related to medications are responsible for 30% of outpatient geriatric consultations and 10–17% of hospital admissions, and it is estimated that over 90% of those admitted have polypharmacy reported [32]. Among the drugs most frequently associated with adverse reactions, warfarin is involved in approximately one-third of these hospitalizations, while insulin, oral antiplatelet agents, and oral hypoglycemic agents accounted for approximately another third. In contrast, medications commonly designated as high risk or potentially inappropriate (according to Beers' generalized criteria) were rarely involved [33, 34].

An adverse reaction to the drug should be suspected whenever an older patient has an unexpected change in their baseline state.

The prevalence of clinically important interactions has been reported to be 15% in a sample of frail older people in the United States [35].

While polypharmacy showed increased mortality in statistical terms [36], the causality of this relationship remains unclear but emphasizes the need for a balanced approach between the risk and benefit of the prescription of medications.

Additionally, polypharmacy is associated with a wide range of clinical consequences, but the risk assessment must be refined, primarily taking into account the "multimorbidity confounder," since the risk is directly related to the comorbidities of the patients and not only with the number of prescribed drugs [37].

Polypharmacy and Frailty

Frailty is a common clinical syndrome in older adults that carries an increased risk for poor health outcomes including falls, incident disability, hospitalization, and mortality [38]. Frailty is theoretically defined as a clinically recognizable state of increased vulnerability resulting from aging-associated decline in reserve and function across multiple physiologic systems, such as when the ability to cope with everyday or acute stressors is comprised. There are two main established methods for the evaluation of frailty: (i) Fried's criteria, which define a clinical syndrome or phenotype, including weight loss, exhaustion, weak grip strength, slow walking speed, and low physical activity, and (ii) the Frailty Index, first developed by Rockwood et al. which counts accumulated deficits of measures such as symptoms, signs, diseases, and disabilities with the hypothesis that the more deficits a person has, the more likely that person is to be frail.

Frailty and polypharmacy are common and widely studied entities in geriatric patients, although little is known about the impact they may have on each other. Undoubtedly, frailty can be observed as a cause of polypharmacy, but it can also be a consequence of polypharmacy and even a risk factor for negative outcomes with regard to drug-drug interaction and adverse drug reactions. Frailty is associated with physiological changes, chronic diseases, a diminished cognitive status, as well as PK/PD changes.

The association between frailty and polypharmacy seems so evident that even some scales or tools to measure frailty, including the Edmonton Frail Scale, the Groningen Frailty Indicator, or some versions of Frailty Index, include the consumption of drugs.

Despite the obvious association, it is difficult to establish causality and determine what occurs first: frailty or polypharmacy.

Observational studies have determined that frail patients are more prone to be under polypharmacy than robust patients and that beyond 6.5 co-prescribed drugs the number of frail patients increases exponentially [39].

Again, we lack prospective studies that can assess the transition to pre-frailty and frailty along with the addition of prescribed drugs to analyze the sequence of events and the relation between frailty and polypharmacy.

Herr et al. showed that excessive polypharmacy and frailty are independent risk factors for mortality, but the combination of both multiplied by 6.30 the risk of dying during a 2.6-year follow-up period [40].

Medicinal Cannabis Use in Older People

As medicinal cannabis gains better regulation from health authorities around the globe, its use increases notoriously. Older people are no exception to this phenomenon, and they certainly take advantage of this alternative. The 2016 National Survey of Drug Use and Health showed a tenfold increase in cannabis use among adults over age 65. Researchers from the University of Colorado conducted a qualitative study about cannabinoid use in older patients, and one of the findings was that patients were reluctant to discuss with their doctors about the use of cannabinoids and that they preferred recreational cannabis instead of medicinal cannabis. The clinical situations in which patients use cannabinoids are generally pain, anxiety, and depression [41].

Health teams must be aware of the use of medicinal cannabis by their patients and ready to deal with side effects, interactions, and, eventually, with abstinence syndrome, especially during hospitalizations.

In general, older patients may be more sensitive to the effects of drugs acting on the CNS. A number of physiological factors may contribute to this sensitivity such as (1) age-related changes in brain volume, number of neurons, and neurotransmitter sensitivity, (2) age-related changes in the pre- and post-synaptic number and sensitivity of neurotransmitter receptors, and (3) changes in drug distribution in older people, with higher concentrations of psychotropic drugs in the CNS [42].

A couple of studies have found that the most reported adverse events related to medicinal cannabis use are sedation-like symptoms, such as drowsiness, tiredness, and somnolence [43, 44]. Nervous system-related adverse events are of particular interest in geriatrics because they increase the risk of falls, which leads to an increased morbidity and mortality. This finding could be of major clinical importance in older patients, as these adverse events may lead to an increased risk of falls, especially when administering higher doses of cannabinoids, as tetrahydrocannabinol (THC) is known to cause a dose-dependent increase in adverse events [45].

However, it is worth noting that cannabinoids have a safety profile that does not raise serious concerns about their use as a general rule. The rate of serious adverse events did not differ significantly between cannabinoid group and controls (RR 1.04, 95% CI 0.78–1.39) in the systematic review performed by Wang et al. [44]. In the systematic review by van den Elsen et al., one serious adverse event was found: the development of a grand mal seizure in an older subject with Alzheimer's disease, directly after receiving 2.5 mg dronabinol [43]. This finding is certainly difficult to interpret as the literature suggests that cannabinoid agonists may actually have an anti-epileptic effect [46].

Older patients treated with cannabinoids have to be strictly assessed and followed up about their cardiovascular system status, as they can experience low blood pressure and cardiac arrhythmias [47].

Cannabinoids may be administered through a great variety of route, that is, oral, sublingual, dermal, smoked, inhaled, etc. The pharmacokinetic profile of THC is highly dependent on the route of administration. Oral and sublingual administration of THC is characterized by a slower absorption than inhaled administration; it also has a more extensive first-pass effect and a lower rate of drug delivery to the brain, probably resulting in fewer and delayed adverse effects [48]. Interestingly, oral administration – possibly the preferred route for older adults – results in relatively high plasma concentrations of the metabolite 11-OH-THC, which in turn contributes to psycho-active symptoms [49].

Drug-drug interactions are mediated by pharmacodynamic and/or pharmacokinetic mechanisms. Cannabis is being used in various forms as crude extracts or purified ingredients (with different THC/cannabinoids ratios); therefore, drug interactions caused by cannabis depend not only on the drugs involved but also the chemical components/profiles of the cannabis preparations used. Among pharmacodynamic interactions, we may observe agonism or antagonism between drugs. One of the most profited pharmacodynamic interactions is the synergistic relation between opioids and cannabinoids for the treatment of severe and chronic pain. With regard to other pharmacodynamic interactions, bidirectional effects may be expected when affecting membrane transporters (P-glycoprotein, breast cancer resistance proteins, and multidrug resistance proteins) and metabolizing enzymes (cytochrome P450 and UDP-glucuronosyltransferases). However clinical effects of these interactions seen in vitro are rare due to redundant mechanisms in the organism. Nevertheless, caution should be taken to closely monitor the responses of cannabis users with certain drugs to guard their safety, especially for older people with chronic diseases or kidney and liver conditions [50].

Deprescribing

Polypharmacy in many cases is a consequence of medications prescribed by various health agents, which sometimes are inappropriate or unnecessary but which in turn, for different reasons, are not suspended.

To avoid this in patients affected by multiple pathologies, it is appropriate to establish treatment priorities and always consider an initial non-pharmacological therapeutic approach (e.g., exercise and weight reduction), this helps to avoid polypharmacy, as well as to monitor the benefits and potential damages of prescription drugs to reduce their adverse effects. If it is necessary to initiate a treatment, it is recommended to start with low doses and slow titration, always considering pharmacological interactions at the time of prescription [30, 51].

Deprescription is the process of planned gradual or supervised reduction or the safe withdrawal of potentially inappropriate medications that may cause harm, either because they no longer have that indication or are no longer beneficial to the patient's pathology.

The purpose of deprescription is to reduce inappropriate polypharmacy and the damage of medications and improve outcomes related to the patient's health.

The best way to deprescribe is to reduce medications one by one, and the whole process requires careful evaluation, effort, commitment, and time. Elimination should be considered after careful evaluation of the patient's general health, therapeutic objectives, compliance with the medication with the current treatment regimen, and the willingness to eliminate the medicine. To achieve this successfully, the elimination process must follow an evidence-based, patient-centered, and team-based approach that involves both health professionals and patients/caregivers to effectively reduce inappropriate use of medicines [52].

The dose reduction is particularly useful in multimorbid older adults with cardiovascular disease and concomitant geriatric conditions such as polypharmacy, frailty, and cognitive dysfunction.

Triggers for deprescribing include present or expected adverse reactions to medications, unnecessary polypharmacy, and the need to align medications with the goals of care when life expectancy is reduced [53].

While the deprescription strategy seems to be ideal, it is not without difficulties. Approximately 25% of the polymedicated population refuses to reduce or suspend medications that were being taken despite the recommendation of their general practitioner, mainly those related to disorders of gastric acid, analgesics, and anti-inflammatories. In turn, inertia, conservatism, and fragmented medical care were the main barriers to refusing deprescription [54].

To avoid these problems and make deprescription a useful and daily tool, it is necessary to establish certain parameters so that the process would be feasible, such as implementing standardized deprescription processes in clinical care in a cost-effective way, involving all (patients, health systems, etc.) throughout the process to achieve positive health and quality-of-life results.

It is necessary to incorporate deprescription in the medical culture. The evidence available so far suggests that dose reduction has potential benefits and seems safe [55].

Conclusion

As we described throughout this chapter, the number of chronic diseases added to the increase in life expectancy leads to a high risk of both prevalent and incident polypharmacy. It is assumed that the more comorbidities a person presents, the greater the number of prescribed drugs; therefore, polypharmacy could be considered a reflection of chronic comorbidities [56]. However, the association between increased drugs and morbidity and mortality only finds clinical significance when the drugs are not adequately indicated.

Currently we still have a long way to go in relation to polypharmacy, starting with a more standardized definition that not only contemplates the number of drugs but also takes into account the characteristics of the patient. We must always keep in mind that the more drugs we prescribe to a patient, the greater the risk of potential harm, which may be given not only by an inappropriate indication but also by the different interactions it could have.

On the other hand, we must always prioritize treatments and participate in therapeutic decisions to patients. The periodic review of therapeutic strategies should include deprescription, thus preventing patients from accumulating medications at each consultation.

Rational prescription, as well as deprescription, seems to be the best remedy against polypharmacy.

References

1. Stockl KM, Le L, Zhang S, Harada AS. Clinical and economic outcomes associated with potentially inappropriate prescribing in the elderly. Am J Manag Care. 2010;16:e1–10.
2. World Health Organization. Informe mundial sobre el envejecimiento y la salud. New York: World Health Organization; 2015. https://apps.who.int/iris/bitstream/handle/10665/186466/9789240694873_eng.pdf?sequence=1.
3. Payne RA. The epidemiology of polypharmacy. Clin Med (Lond). 2016;16(5):465–9. https://doi.org/10.7861/clinmedicine.16-5-465.

4. Grimmsmann T, Himmel W. Polypharmacy in primary care practices: an analysis using a large health insurance database. Pharmacoepidemiol Drug Saf. 2009;18(12):1206–13.
5. Alejandro Castro-Rodríguez J, Orozco-Hernández JP, Marín-Medina DS. Polifarmacia y prescripción de medicamentos potencialmente no apropiados en ancianos. Rev Méd Risaralda. 2016;22(1):52–7.
6. Morin L, et al. The epidemiology of polypharmacy in older adults: register-based prospective cohort study. Clin Epidemiol. 2018;10:289–98.
7. Lu W-H, et al. Effect of polypharmacy, potentially inappropriate medications and anticholinergic burden on clinical outcomes: a retrospective cohort study. CMAJ. 2015;187(4):E130–7.
8. Goldberg RM, Mabee J, Chan L, et al. Drug-drug and drug-disease interactions in the ED: analysis of a high-risk population. Am J Emerg Med. 1996;14:447–50.
9. Hajjar ER, et al. Polypharmacy in elderly patients. Am J Geriatr Pharmacother. 2007;5(4):345–51. https://doi.org/10.1016/j.amjopharm.2007.12.002.
10. Kuschel BM, Laflamme L, Möller J. The risk of fall injury in relation to commonly prescribed medications among older people—a Swedish case-control study. Eur J Public Health. 2015;25(3):527–32. https://doi.org/10.1093/eurpub/cku120.
11. Huang AR, Mallet L, Rochefort CM, Eguale T, Buckeridge DL, Tamblyn R. Medication-related falls in the elderly: causative factors and preventive strategies. Drugs Aging. 2012;29(5):359–76. https://doi.org/10.2165/11599460-000000000-00000.
12. Kaufmann CP, et al. Inappropriate prescribing: a systematic overview of published assessment tools. Eur J Clin Pharmacol. 2014;70:1–11.
13. Bressler R, Bahl JJ. Principles of drug therapy for the elderly patient. Mayo Clin Proc. 2003;78(12):1564–77.
14. Musso CG. Acute renal failure in the elderly: pearls for its assessment and treatment. Electron J Biomed. 2005;1:1–93. Renkke H, Denker B. Renal pathophysiology. Philadelphia: Lippincott Williams & Wilkins, 2007.
15. Fulop T Jr, Worum I, Csongor J, Foris G, Leovey A. Body composition in elderly people I. Determination of body composition by multiisotope method and the elimination kinetics of these isotopes in healthy elderly subjects. Gerontology. 1985;31(1):6–14.
16. Ginsberg G, Hattis D, Russ A, Sonawane B. Pharmacokinetic and pharmacodynamic factors that can affect sensitivity to neurotoxic sequelae in elderly individuals. Environ Health Perspect. 2005;113(9):1243–9.
17. McLean AJ, Le Couteur DG. Aging biology and geriatric clinical pharmacology. Pharmacol Rev. 2004;56(2):163–84. Perucca E. Age-related changes in pharmacokinetics: predictability and assessment methods. Int Rev Neurobiol. 2007;81:183–99.
18. Noreddin AM, Haynes V. Use of pharmacodynamic principles to optimise dosage regimens for antibacterial agents in the elderly. Drugs Aging. 2007;24(4):275–92.
19. Mangoni AA, Jackson SH. Age-related changes in pharmacokinetics and pharmacodynamics: basic principles and practical applications. Br J Clin Pharmacol. 2004;57(1):6–14.
20. Zoli M, Magalotti D, Bianchi G, Gueli C, Orlandini C, Grimaldi M, et al. Total and functional hepatic blood flow decrease in parallel with ageing. Age Ageing. 1999;28(1):29–33.
21. Young LL, Lyon CE. Effect of postchill aging and sodium tripolyphosphate on moisture binding properties, color, and Warner-Bratzler shear values of chicken breast meat. Poult Sci. 1997;76(11):1587–90.
22. Wetzels JF, Kiemeney LA, Swinkels DW, Willems HL, den Heijer M. Age- and gender-specific reference values of estimated GFR in Caucasians: the Nijmegen Biomedical Study. Kidney Int. 2007;72(5):632–7.
23. Lindeman RD, Tobin J, Shock NW. Longitudinal studies on the rate of decline in renal function with age. J Am Geriatr Soc. 1985;33(4):278–85.
24. Delafuente JC. Pharmacokinetic and pharmacodynamic alterations in the geriatric patient. Consult Pharm. 2008;23(4):324–34.
25. Waltman KWS, editor. Preventing adverse drug reactions. Philadelphia: Hanley & Belfus; 2000.

26. Catterson ML, Preskorn SH, Martin RL. Pharmacodynamic and pharmacokinetic considerations in geriatric psychopharmacology. Psychiatr Clin North Am. 1997;20(1):205–18.
27. Dettli L. Drug dosage in renal disease. Clin Pharmacokinet. 1976;1(2):126–34.
28. Abernethy DR. Aging effects on drug disposition and effect. Geriatr Nephrol Urol. 1999;9(1):15–9.
29. Gardiner SJ, Begg EJ. Pharmacogenetics, drug-metabolizing enzymes, and clinical practice. Pharmacol Rev. 2006;58(3):521–90.
30. Denneboom W, Dautzenberg MG, Grol R, De Smet PA. Analysis of polypharmacy in older patients in primary care using a multidisciplinary expert panel. Br J Gen Pract. 2006;56(528):504–10.
31. Ghiculescu R. Therapeutic drug monitoring: which drugs, why, when and how to do it. Aust Prescr. 2008;31(2):42–4.
32. Pedrós C, Formiga F, Corbella X, Arnau JM. Adverse drug reactions leading to urgent hospital admission in an elderly population: prevalence and main features. Eur J Clin Pharmacol. 2016;72:219–26. https://doi.org/10.1007/s00228-015-1974-0.
33. American Geriatrics Society 2012 Beers Criteria Update Expert Panel. American Geriatrics Society updated Beers Criteria for potentially inappropriate medication use in older adults. J Am Geriatr Soc. 2012;60(4):616–31.
34. Budnitz DS, Shehab N, Kegler SR, Richards CL. Medication use leading to emergency department visits for adverse drug events in older adults. Ann Intern Med. 2007;147(11):755–65.
35. Lindblad CI, et al. Clinically important drug disease interactions and their prevalence in older adults. Clin Ther. 2006;28(8):1133–43.
36. Leelakanok N, Holcombe AL, Lund BC, Xiaomei G, Schweizer ML. Association between polypharmacy and death: a systematic review and meta-analysis. J Am Pharm Assoc. 2017;57(6):729–738.e10.
37. Wastesson JW, Morin L, Tan ECK, Johnell K. An update on the clinical consequences of polypharmacy in older adults: a narrative review. Expert Opin Drug Saf. 2018;17(12):1185–96.
38. Xue Q-L. The frailty syndrome: definition and natural history. Clin Geriatr Med. 2011;27(1):1–15.
39. Corsonello A, et al. Polypharmacy in elderly patients at discharge from the acute care hospital. Ther Clin Risk Manag. 2007;3(1):197–203.
40. Herr M, et al. Polypharmacy and frailty: prevalence, relationship, and impact on mortality in a French sample of 2350 old people. Pharmacoepidemiol Drug Saf. 2015;24(6):637–46.
41. Bobitt J, et al. Qualitative analysis of cannabis use among older adults in Colorado. Drugs Aging. 2019;36(7):655–66. https://doi.org/10.1007/s40266-019-00665-w.
42. Canada H. Information for healthcare professionals on cannabis and the cannabinoids. Ottawa: Health Canada; 2018. ISBN: 978-0-660-27828-5.
43. van den Elsen GA, et al. Efficacy and safety of medical cannabinoids in older subjects: a systematic review. Ageing Res Rev. 2014;14:56–64.
44. Wang T, Collet JP, Shapiro S, Ware MA. Adverse effects of medical cannabinoids: a systematic review. Can Med Assoc J. 2008;178:1669–78.
45. Mizrahi R, et al. Mechanisms contributing to cognitive deficits in cannabis users. Neuropharmacology. 2017;124:84–8.
46. Gloss D, Vickrey B. Cannabinoids for epilepsy (review). Cochrane Database Syst Rev. 2014;(3):CD009270.
47. Randall MD, et al. Cardiovascular effects of cannabinoids. Pharmacol Ther. 2002;95(2):191–202.
48. Karschner EL, et al. Predictive model accuracy in estimating last Δ9-tetrahydrocannabinol (THC) intake from plasma and whole blood cannabinoid concentrations in chronic, daily cannabis smokers administered subchronic oral THC. Drug Alcohol Depend. 2012;125(3):313–9.
49. Klumpers LE, et al. Manipulating brain connectivity with δ^9-tetrahydrocannabinol: a pharmacological resting state FMRI study. NeuroImage. 2012;63(3):1701–11.

50. Alsherbiny MA, et al. Medicinal cannabis—potential drug interactions. Medicines (Basel). 2019;6(1):3.
51. Butler JM, Begg EJ. Free drug metabolic clearance in elderly people. Clin Pharmacokinet. 2008;47(5):297–321.
52. Salahudeen MS. Deprescribing medications in older people: a narrative review. Drugs Today (Barc). 2018;54(8):489–98. https://doi.org/10.1358/dot.2018.54.8.2856495.
53. Krishnaswami A, et al. Deprescribing in older adults with cardiovascular disease. J Am Coll Cardiol. 2019;73(20):2584–95. https://doi.org/10.1016/j.jacc.2019.03.467.
54. Zechmann S, Trueb C, Valeri F, Streit S, Senn O, Neuner-Jehle S. Barriers and enablers for deprescribing among older, multimorbid patients with polypharmacy: an explorative study from Switzerland. BMC Fam Pract. 2019;20(1):64. https://doi.org/10.1186/s12875-019-0953-4.
55. Reeve E, Thompson W, Farrell B. Deprescribing: a narrative review of the evidence and practical recommendations for recognizing opportunities and taking action. Eur J Intern Med. 2017;38:3–11. https://doi.org/10.1016/j.ejim.2016.12.021. Epub 2017 Jan 5.
56. Cadogan CA, Ryan C, Hughes CM. Appropriate polypharmacy and medicine safety: when many is not too many. Drug Saf. 2016;39(2):109–16.

Chapter 8
Vitamin D and Frailty

Jack Feehan, Steven Phu, and Gustavo Duque

Introduction

Since its discovery shortly after the turn of the twentieth century, the scientific understanding of the physiology of vitamin D has evolved significantly [1] from a vitamin with a role in bone health and prevention of rickets to the complex hormone that it is now understood to be. Indeed, its importance across a wide range of areas is becoming clear. Vitamin D is a critical mediator between the musculoskeletal and renal systems, and an understanding of how it affects and in turn is affected by each of these systems in the development of frailty is key to the management of geriatric patients into the future. In this chapter, we summarize current evidence on the role of vitamin D in physical and cognitive frailty and updated recommendations on vitamin D supplementation in frail older patients.

J. Feehan · G. Duque (✉)
Australian Institute for Musculoskeletal Science (AIMSS), The University of Melbourne and Western Health, St. Albans, VIC, Australia

Department of Medicine-Western Health, The University of Melbourne, St. Albans, VIC, Australia
e-mail: gustavo.duque@unimelb.edu.au

S. Phu
Department of Medicine-Western Health, The University of Melbourne, St. Albans, VIC, Australia

Falls, Balance and Injury Research Centre, Neuroscience Research Australia, University of New South Wales, Sydney, NSW, Australia

© Springer Nature Switzerland AG 2021

C. G. Musso et al. (eds.), *Frailty and Kidney Disease*,
https://doi.org/10.1007/978-3-030-53529-2_8

Vitamin D: Biosynthesis, Action, and Metabolism

Vitamin D refers to a group of fat-soluble secosteroids, with a wide range of actions across multiple tissues and physiologies [2]. While referred to as vitamins, these compounds are more correctly endocrine hormones in terms of their physiological nature and effects [3]. Vitamin D is gained in small quantities from the diet (particularly in foods fortified with vitamin D) or from supplementation, however sun exposure is the major source in humans (Fig. 8.1). While there are a number of members of this group, the most biologically relevant is cholecalciferol, also commonly known as vitamin D_3, which is principally synthesized when the deeper layers of the dermis are exposed to sunlight. Other members of the vitamin D superfamily which have small but still relevant effects include ergocalciferol (or vitamin D_2) [4].

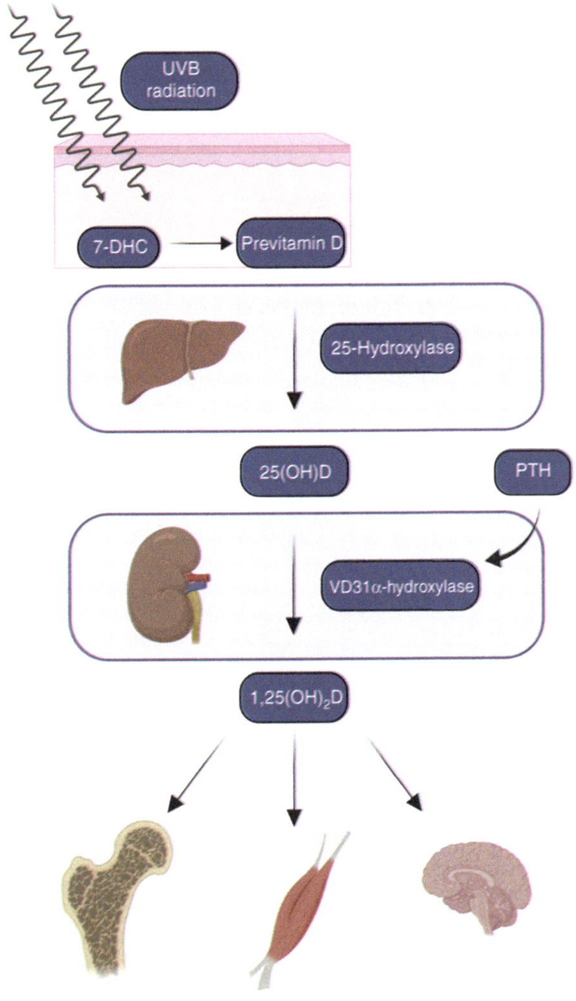

Fig. 8.1 Vitamin D metabolism and clinical effects related to frailty

Cholecalciferol is an inactive prohormone, requiring a two-step process of hydroxylation before it becomes the biologically active form of vitamin D, calcitriol. The kidney plays a key role in the activation and regulation of vitamin D, and alterations to renal function have a profound impact on the biological activity of this hormone.

Biosynthesis (Fig. 8.1)

Vitamin D synthesis begins with the photoisomerization of 7-dehydrocholesterol (7-DHC) in the deeper layers of the epidermis, particularly in the stratum basale and stratum spinosum [5]. The origin of 7-DHC in the epidermis is not fully understood. It was once thought to be transported from the epithelial layers of the digestive tract, but has been shown in high concentrations in the membranes of epidermal keratinocytes, and is likely to be secreted from the skin itself as part of the pathway of cholesterol synthesis. 7-DHC is a photo acceptor of UVB radiation, absorbing light 290–320 nm range with a peak production range between 295 and 300 nm [6]. On exposure to radiation in these ranges, chemical bonds are broken in the hydrocarbon ring, causing it to open, becoming pre-vitamin D, which rapidly undergoes spontaneous isomerization to form cholecalciferol [6]. Once synthesized, cholecalciferol circulates until it reaches the liver, where it undergoes its first hydroxylation by the vitamin D 25-hydroxylase enzyme in the hepatocyte to form 25-hydroxyvitamin D (25(OH)D) or calcifediol [7]. Calcifediol has a long half-life (19–29 days), which makes it an effective reservoir for vitamin D in the circulation, where it remains as an inactive precursor hormone [8]. When required, calcifediol is activated in the proximal tubule of the nephron, where it undergoes a second hydroxylation by the enzyme 25-hydroxyvitamin D_3 1-alpha-hydroxylase (VD31A), becoming the biologically active hormone, calcitriol, or 1,25-hydroxyvitamin D [9]. In contrast to calcifediol, calcitriol has a very short life span (5–8 h) but has a significantly stronger affinity for the vitamin D receptor (VDR) and subsequently a much larger biological effect in the target tissues [10].

The final step in vitamin D activation by the kidney also serves as the key regulation point for its metabolism and action. In response to decreased serum concentrations of calcium, parathyroid hormone (PTH) is released. As well as acting directly on the receptor activator of nuclear factor κB ligand (RANKL)/osteoprotegerin (OPG) axis to increase release of calcium from the skeleton [11], it acts to upregulate the activity of the VD31A enzyme in the renal tubules, causing more activation of vitamin D [12]. It is also of note that as concentrations of calcitriol increase, the release of PTH's antagonist hormone calcitonin is inhibited [13].

Biological Activity

The biological effects of vitamin D are largely attributed to its binding of the VDR. The VDR is expressed in a wide range of cell types and unbound is located in the cytosol [14]. Once the fat-soluble, active vitamin D diffuses into the cell, it binds to the VDR in the cytosol and translocates to the nucleus. Here the receptor-ligand complex acts as a transcription factor, increasing expression of effector proteins specific to the tissue in which it is acting [14]. The VDR is involved in the regulation of a large array of functions, causing changes in the expression of over 900 genes in humans across a broad range of physiological systems and pathways [15].

While calcitriol has a wide spectrum of biological effects, its role in mineral homeostasis is the most well defined. Calcitriol strongly increases circulating concentrations of calcium, via three major mechanisms, acting on the intestinal mucosa to increase Ca^{2+} absorption, on the renal tubules to increase reabsorption, and on the bone to promote mineral release. In all three of these mechanisms, it acts in synergy with PTH.

In the intestinal mucosa, activation of the VDR causes an increase in the synthesis of calcium-binding protein. This causes increased capacity of the epithelial cells in the intestinal mucosa to bind to and absorb calcium in the gastrointestinal tract, increasing uptake from the diet [16]. This effect is mirrored in the renal tubules, with increased expression of calcium-binding protein in both the proximal and distal tubules, causing increased reabsorption [17]. Finally, vitamin D acts on the osteoblast, causing an increase in the expression of the receptor activator of nuclear factor kappa-B ligand (RANKL), which acts to increase osteoclastogenesis [18]. The pro-resorptive effect of vitamin D appears counterintuitive, given the well-known associations of deficiency with conditions such as rickets, osteomalacia, and osteoporosis. It is believed that this discrepancy is caused by the strong effect vitamin D has on intestinal absorption, which results in a net gain in calcium, the excess of which is later incorporated into the bone.

Outside mineral homeostasis, vitamin D has a number of other biological effects relevant to the onset of kidney disease and frailty. VDR is expressed in skeletal muscle, and vitamin D regulates gene expression and modulates ligand-dependent uptake of 25-hydroxyvitamin D3 in primary myofibers thus acting as a myotrophic factor [10]. In addition, it has also shown to be strongly anti-inflammatory, with the activation of the VDR inducing decreased cytokine secretion, inhibiting activity of both innate and acquired immune cells, as well as downregulating activity of several other key inflammatory pathways [19]. There is also mounting evidence that vitamin D has a role in inhibiting the renin-angiotensin system. Vitamin D acts to inhibit the activity of renin, and subsequently decrease the levels of angiotensin II in the circulation, providing a protective benefit in hypertensive disease [20].

Vitamin D Deficiency in Kidney Disease (Fig. 8.2)

Vitamin D metabolism is strongly influenced by the kidney and in turn has strong effects on renal physiology. Any renal pathology that results in diminished glomerular filtration rate (GFR), particularly in a chronic setting, will cause vitamin D deficiency [9].

One of the major drivers in this deficiency centers on the key activation step of vitamin D by the VD31A enzyme in the proximal renal tubular epithelium.

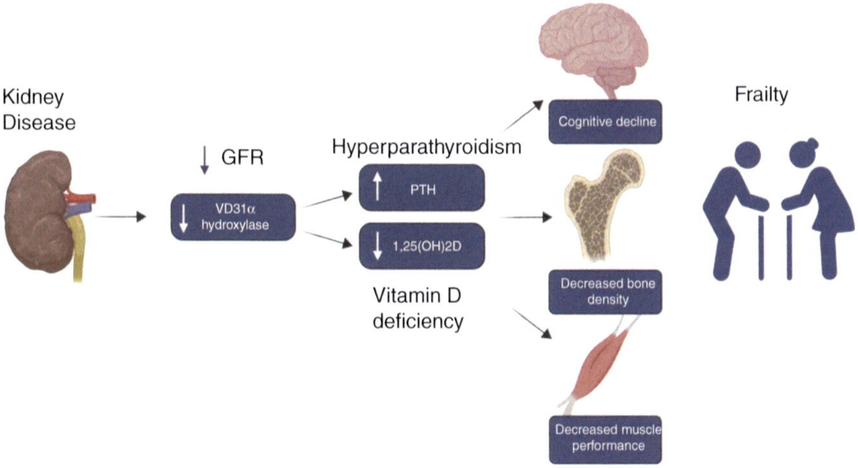

Fig. 8.2 Relationship between vitamin D deficiency features, sarcopenia, and frailty

As mounting kidney damage occurs, the resulting decrease in GFR causes diminished exposure of vitamin D to the enzyme with a corresponding decrease in activation [21]. This leads to a functional loss of vitamin D, as it becomes "trapped" in its inactive precursor form. This ongoing vitamin D deficiency causes a progressive decline in serum calcium concentration due to compromised intestinal absorption, with corresponding increases in PTH secretion to counter this. However as the action of PTH is partly vitamin D dependant, secondary hyperparathyroidism occurs. This increase in PTH levels as a result of vitamin D deficiency is a recognized cause of secondary hyperparathyroidism [22].

This chronic elevation of PTH contributes to the onset of frailty, particularly from the perspective of weakening bone and muscle. As vitamin D-mediated intestinal calcium absorption is compromised, serum concentrations of calcium must be maintained through bone resorption. As mentioned earlier, ordinarily the action of PTH on bone resorption is countered by the significantly larger influx of calcium from the gastrointestinal tract. However as the intestinal response is vitamin D dependant, it no longer occurs, or is compromised, and so bone quality is diminished over time [22, 23]. The role of secondary hyperparathyroidism in the extra-skeletal components of frailty is still unclear; however, a number of studies have shown a correlation between the two. Increased PTH levels are associated with both incidence of frailty [24] and reduced gait velocity, grip strength, and limits of stability in older persons [24].

In summary, kidney disease is an important cause of vitamin D deficiency, and an understanding of the underlying mechanisms behind this is vital in the treatment of these patients. Ongoing deficiency, associated with alterations in the target tissues combined with elevated serum PTH, has a large impact on overall condition of the patient, with a steady decline into frailty commonly occurring as a result.

Vitamin D Deficiency: Clinical Manifestations

As described above, vitamin D is metabolized through several processes with the assistance and feedback of hormones such as parathyroid hormone (PTH). In recent times, identification of the presence of the VDR in other tissues such as in the muscular and nervous systems has resulted in increased interest in the outcomes associated with vitamin D deficiency.

Epidemiology of Vitamin D Deficiency

The gold standard of vitamin D assessment is the measurement of 25(OH)D concentration, the inactive precursor form of vitamin D, due to its stability and long half-life [25]. Deficient levels of vitamin D are defined as those less than 50 nmol/L (20 ng/mL), with individuals presenting with levels below 30 nmol/L (12 ng/mL) considered severely deficient with increasing risk of osteomalacia (defined as the presence of higher amount of unmineralized bone matrix) or rickets [26, 27]. However the limits are difficult to define due to the drastic seasonal changes in circulating vitamin D due to changes in sun exposure [28]. Epidemiological studies have found significant numbers of vitamin D deficiency across multiple populations of older adults, with prevalence ranging from 17.4% to as high as 70.7% [29–32].

With regard to frailty, there is strong evidence highlighting the links between vitamin D status and frailty. When classifying those who presented with adequate and inadequate levels of vitamin D using a cut-point of 75 nmol/L (30 ng/mL) in Korean older adults aged 70–84 years, an increased likelihood of frailty was found [33]. In another study comparing Italian men and women over the age of 65 years, those who were vitamin D-deficient (<50 nmol/L) were significantly more likely to present with frailty with odds ratios of 4.94 and 1.43, respectively [34]. In a prospective study which followed older women from the ages of 75–85 years, associations were also evident between vitamin D deficiency (levels below 50 nmol/L) at 80 years and future frailty [35]. Finally, a study of Portuguese older adults presenting with vitamin D levels in the lowest quartile consistent with severe deficiency (<30 nmol/L or 12 ng/mL) has identified significantly increased risk of pre-frailty (2.65 times more likely) and frailty (3.77 times more likely) [36]. These studies provide strong evidence for the role of vitamin D deficiency in frailty. With an aging population worldwide, the prevalence of vitamin D deficiency and frailty is expected to increase, placing considerable strain on healthcare systems [37].

There are a number of important risk factors for vitamin D deficiency. Studies have reported links between low sun exposure [29, 31, 32], older age [29, 31, 33], physical inactivity [31, 32], socioeconomic status [29, 31, 32], smoking [31], obesity [31], living alone [31], and darker skin tone [30] with vitamin D deficiency. Importantly many of these risk factors also coincide with those of frailty [38], and vitamin D deficiency commonly presents with a multitude of varied clinical manifestations.

Clinical Manifestations

The identification of the VDR located in numerous organs and tissues has resulted in numerous studies examining the role of vitamin D deficiency on bodily functions across a number of physiologies, including the musculoskeletal, cardiovascular, nervous, and immune systems. This section will focus on the impact of vitamin D deficiencies which directly contribute to the development of frailty, in particular, bone, muscle, and cognitive function.

Bone and Fractures

As the primary role of vitamin D is to maintain calcium homeostasis, dysregulation of this system due to low reserves of vitamin D has profound impacts on the bone [39]. These effects were evident in a large Dutch study of over 1000 older adults, with vitamin D-deficient participants expressing a combination of increased bone turnover, lower bone mineral density, and increased PTH levels [40]. Interestingly, bone mineral density and total bone mineral content were found to increase consistently until levels of 50–60 nmol/L were achieved, further highlighting the interactions between vitamin D and bone. Left untreated, long-term vitamin D deficiency and the resulting hyperparathyroidism may lead to the development of osteomalacia and osteoporosis which are both characterized by the weakening of bone, thereby increasing the risk of fractures. Evidence of this has been shown in work by van Schoor and Heymans [41], where older adults between the ages of 65 and 75 years with severe deficiency in vitamin D (<30 nmol/L) presented with more than three times increased risk of fractures over the course of a 6-year follow-up compared to those with vitamin D levels >30 nmol/L. However, not only were participants in this study at increased risk for fractures, but significantly increased risk for falls (4.5 times more likely) and poor physical performance (1.5 times more likely) were also evident and will be discussed in upcoming sections.

Finally, it is important to consider the wider implications of vitamin D-related declines in both health, particularly regarding osteoporosis. Osteoporosis has been shown to have a direct relationship with frailty incidence in Japanese older adults, increasing the likelihood of frailty development over a 4-year period by more than threefold [42].

Muscle and Falls

Given the expression of the VDR in muscle, numerous studies have been performed to examine the impact of vitamin D deficiency on muscle outcomes (strength, performance, gait, and balance) which are associated with falls risk. In a study of Italian older adults, severe deficiency in vitamin D levels (<25 nmol/L) was significantly associated with poorer performance in the Short Physical Performance Battery (SPPB), an assessment tool comprising measures of balance, strength, and mobility [43]. Muscle strength too, measured by handgrip strength, was significantly reduced in those presenting with deficient levels (<50 nmol/L) of vitamin D. Similar to the findings of vitamin D deficiency in bone, PTH was identified as a potential mediator of these associations in this study [43]. Findings of poor strength and physical performance have also been shown in an English population aged 60 years and above where over 25% of older adults who were severely vitamin D-deficient (<30 nmol/L) presented with low performance in the SPPB (score ≤ 6) and over 40% presented with low handgrip strength categorized using sarcopenia guidelines [44]. The longitudinal effects of vitamin D deficiency on physical performance have also been shown in a study of Dutch older adults, where significant declines in physical performance over a 3-year period were associated with vitamin D levels below 20 ng/mL (50 nmol/L) [45]. Interestingly, further analysis of this cohort reported a steady increase in physical performance measures occurring with every 10 nmol/L increase in vitamin D levels, which stabilized once levels >50 nmol/L were reached [41]. These findings were similar to that discussed in the previous section regarding bone mineral density.

Gait speed, considered by some to be the sixth vital sign due to its relationship with a diverse range of adverse outcomes in frail older persons [46], has also shown a strong relationship with vitamin D deficiency [47, 48]. In a recent systematic review and meta-analysis, gait speed was both statistically and clinically different between vitamin D-deficient and vitamin D-sufficient older adults by up to 0.18 m/s [47]. Baseline vitamin D levels were also found to be associated with greater declines in gait speed. Postural control and balance are also negatively impacted with vitamin D deficiency, with declines in stability and postural control observed [48, 49]. When combined with the aforementioned declines in muscle strength, physical performance, and gait, an increased risk of falls will be present in vitamin D-deficient older adults.

Differences in muscle and performance components related to vitamin D deficiency also exist within categories of frailty. In a study including 127 pre-frail and frail older adults where 53% presented with vitamin D deficiency, impairments in physical performance (SPPB) were noted in addition to reduced appendicular lean mass [50]. Therefore, the findings of detrimental effects of vitamin D deficiency on measures of muscle strength, mass, and physical performance should also be considered in the context of sarcopenia. Sarcopenia is classified as the presence of low muscle strength, mass, and poor physical performance resulting in adverse outcomes [51] such as nearly twofold increased risk of falls and fractures [52]. Furthermore, as sarcopenia components and outcomes coincide with that of physical frailty [53], declines in muscle strength and physical performance in at-risk

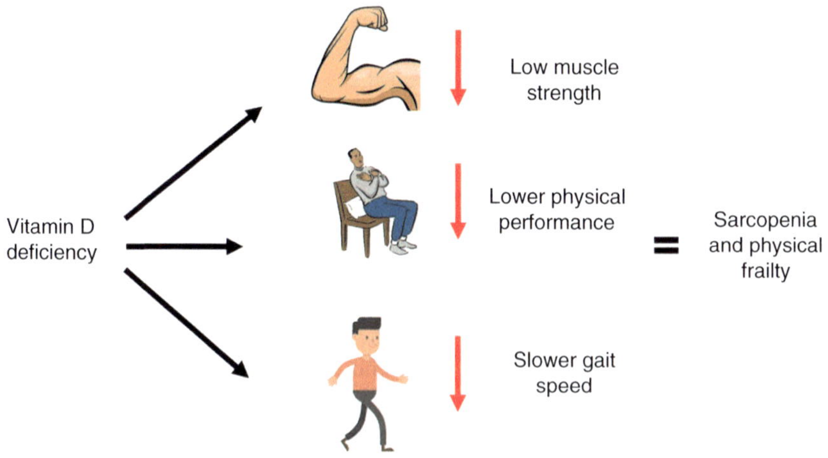

Fig. 8.3 Impact of vitamin D supplementation dose on falls and fracture outcomes

older adults presenting with vitamin D deficiency highlight the need for early interventions (Fig. 8.3).

Vitamin D, Cognition, and Cognitive Frailty

With findings of VDR in the nervous system, there has been a suggestion that vitamin D deficiency may impact cognitive function in older adults with mixed findings in literature. In a large study of more than 3000 older adults in the United States, an increased likelihood of impairment in various components of cognitive function was evident across the vitamin D-deficient and severely deficient [54]. Vitamin D-deficient older adults were 1.4 times more likely to present with cognitive impairments, whereas the severely deficient presented with a 3.9 times increased likelihood of cognitive impairment after adjusting for confounders. These findings were in agreement with a systematic review and meta-analysis where vitamin D-deficient older adults performed worse in the Mini-Mental State Examination (MMSE) and were more likely to present with Alzheimer's disease [55]. Longitudinally, a 5-year follow-up study conducted in Korean older adults found severe vitamin D deficiencies at baseline to be independently predictive of progressive declines in cognitive function and development of mild cognitive impairments [56]. However, it is important to note that these participants may have initially presented with risk of cognitive impairments, with MMSE scores below 27. These findings contrast with more recent work from Lee et al. [57] who only reported significant associations between vitamin D status and cognition when unadjusted for confounders. However, it is important to note that participants in this study were only grouped into sufficient and insufficient levels using a cut-point of 30 ng/mL (75 nmol/L) for analysis.

Vitamin D deficiency in older adults presents a great challenge for healthcare professionals given its high prevalence and diverse clinical manifestations. Vitamin D-deficient older adults may present with a diverse range of signs and symptoms ranging from low bone mineral density to muscular weakness, poor balance, and cognitive difficulties which coincide with that of frailty. Sarcopenia and osteoporosis should also be considered in vitamin D-deficient older adults and predispose to frailty and resulting adverse outcomes such as falls, fractures, disability, and loss of independence.

Vitamin D as a Therapy for Frailty (Fig. 8.3)

Despite knowledge of the adverse effects of vitamin deficiency on general health and well-being, there is limited literature examining the effect of vitamin D supplementation on preventing/treating frailty. In a recent systematic review and dose-response analysis, it was suggested that an increase of 25 nmol/L, equivalent to an intake of 1000 IU of vitamin D3, may reduce the incidence of frailty by 11% [58]. This was in contrast with a large study assessing vitamin D supplementation over 8 years which reported no changes in frailty risk [59]. However, a significant limitation commonly reported in studies performing interventions with vitamin D supplementation is that vitamin D status is not assessed. Therefore, it is often unclear what the true effects of supplementation on vitamin D-deficient participants are. Another important consideration when using vitamin D as therapy for frailty are the diverse risk factors. Given the multitude of risk factors for frailty, interventions are often required to be multidisciplinary, targeting a combination of dietary and lifestyle factors. Although studies performed using vitamin D as a primary intervention for frailty are lacking, numerous studies assessing the effect of vitamin D supplementation on components and outcomes of frailty including muscle strength, physical performance, balance, gait, falls, and fractures exist.

Muscle Strength, Physical Performance, and Balance

Vitamin D supplementation has consistently shown benefits in muscle parameters, particularly strength, which may play a significant role in treating frail older adults. In a meta-analysis performed in 2011 assessing the effect of vitamin D on muscle strength, gait, and balance, significant declines in postural sway and time to complete the Timed Up and Go test were found, in addition to small increases in muscle strength with daily doses of 800–1000 IU/day [60]. Importantly, high single doses did not achieve consistent improvements in physical performance, with the authors suggesting smaller doses taken daily were optimal. Baseline levels of vitamin D should also be taken into consideration with another study only reporting improvements in lower limb muscle strength in participants presenting with vitamin D levels less than 25 nmol/L [61].

The importance of vitamin D supplementation in improving musculoskeletal outcomes has also been reported in multidisciplinary interventions including exercise and/or nutrition. In a meta-analysis of studies on resistance training and vitamin D interventions, an additive effect was found for vitamin D supplementation in improving lower limb strength [62]. However, in contrast to other studies, no additional benefit was reported for physical performance measures. Again, the additive benefit was only attributed to vitamin D-deficient participants. Vitamin D supplementation may also play an important role in nutritional interventions for sarcopenia and frailty, with the PROVIDE study finding participants with baseline vitamin D above deficient levels (>50 nmol/L) achieved the greatest increases in muscle mass after a 13-week intervention [63].

Falls and Fractures

Investigations of the role of vitamin D supplementation in falls prevention have resulted in conflicting results, primarily due to the characteristics of study participants. For example, a Cochrane review performed assessing the interventions for preventing falls in community-dwelling older adults as group did not find any significant effect [64]. However, subgroup analysis of studies conducted in vitamin D-deficient older adults found a significant reduction in the rate and risk for falls, again highlighting the importance of supplementation for deficient individuals. These findings were consistent with that of an earlier meta-analysis which reported significant declines in falls rates by up to 26% within 2–5 months using a dose of 700–1000 IU [65]. These positive results achieved by vitamin D repletion in older adults may in part be attributed to the previously mentioned benefits in muscle strength and balance.

Given the primary role of vitamin D in the maintenance of calcium homeostasis and bone diseases associated with severe deficiencies in vitamin D, the effect of vitamin D supplementation for fracture prevention has been well studied. However, similar to studies in falls, mixed findings were reported due to methodological limitations. In a recent systematic review evaluating the effect of vitamin D, calcium, and combined supplementation as a primary intervention for fracture prevention, the authors concluded that vitamin D supplementation alone did not reduce fracture incidence. However, it was also stated that it was unknown whether participants were vitamin D-deficient, were osteoporotic, or reported previous fractures [66]. In contrast to this, earlier work suggested that supplementation of 700–800 IU/day of vitamin D reduced the relative risk of hip and nonvertebral fractures [67]. It is also important to note that for fracture prevention, particularly in osteoporotic older adults, a diverse range of effective pharmacological therapies are available. As such,

Fig. 8.4 Recommended dosing of vitamin D in vitamin D-deficient and high-risk populations. Doses <800 are ineffective, whereas doses >4000 IU/day or large loading doses increase the risk of falls and fractures

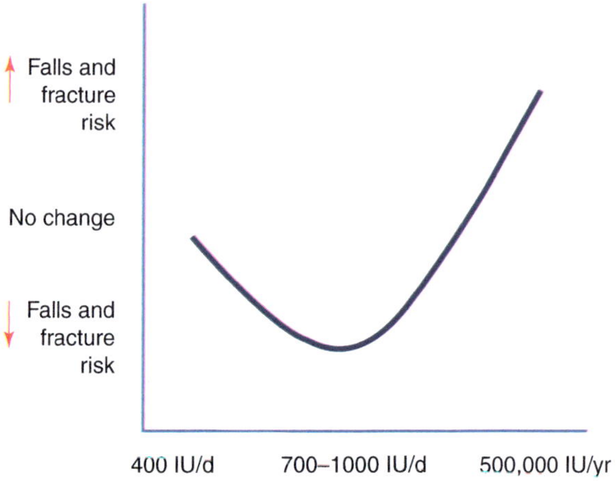

the supplementation of vitamin D to achieve sufficient levels contributes in part to more targeted interventions such as antiresorptives and bone anabolic agents.

Finally, it is important to discuss the dosage of vitamin D supplementation for falls and fracture prevention (Fig. 8.4). While studies reported in this section have typically employed doses of 700–1000 IU for both falls and fracture prevention, the use of a high single yearly dose of 500,000 IU is not recommended and has in fact shown significant detrimental effects. In an Australian study of more than 2000 women aged 70 years and over, randomized to receive a single high dose of vitamin D, the supplementation group surprisingly reported a significantly increased incidence of both falls and fractures compared to the control group [68].

While there is currently limited evidence for the use of vitamin D as the primary intervention for frailty given the numerous risk factors, vitamin D supplementation has been shown to independently improve frailty components and outcomes. There is consistent evidence suggesting vitamin D supplementations of 1000 IU/day are able to improve muscle parameters, falls, and fractures in deficient populations. Larger single doses are not recommended and have been found to be detrimental for falls and fracture prevention.

Conclusion

Solid evidence supports a pivotal role of vitamin D in the physiology of multiple organs and systems. Frailty affects several organs that require physiological levels of vitamin D including bone, muscle, and brain. Low-serum vitamin D is associated with adverse outcomes (i.e., falls, fractures, decreased functional status), which are highly prevalent in frail older persons. Secondary hyperparathyroidism could worsen these manifestations. Due to its high prevalence in this population, serum vitamin D quantification should be a regular practice in frail older patients. Supplementation of

≥800 IU of vitamin D together with ≥1000 mg of calcium reduces the risk for hip fractures and all non-vertebral fractures by about 20%. It also decreases falls risk by approximately 20%. In patients with apparent vitamin D deficiency, normal serum 25(OH)D levels should be restored and maintained using evidence-based recommended dosing. Overall, normalizing serum vitamin D in frail older persons has well-demonstrated beneficial effects on multiple outcomes and should be an integral element of any multidimensional approach in this population.

References

1. Bouillon R, Okamura WH, Norman AW. Structure-function relationships in the vitamin D endocrine system*. Endocr Rev. 1995;16(2):200–57.
2. Holick MF. Sunlight and vitamin D for bone health and prevention of autoimmune diseases, cancers, and cardiovascular disease. Am J Clin Nutr. 2004;80(6):1678S–88S.
3. Norman AW. From vitamin D to hormone D: fundamentals of the vitamin D endocrine system essential for good health. Am J Clin Nutr. 2008;88(2):491S–9S.
4. Nigwekar SU, Bhan I, Thadhani R. Ergocalciferol and cholecalciferol in CKD. Am J Kidney Dis. 2012;60(1):139–56.
5. Holick M, Frommer J, McNeill S, Richtand N, Henley J, Potts J Jr. Photometabolism of 7-dehydrocholesterol to previtamin D3 in skin. Biochem Biophys Res Commun. 1977;76(1):107–14.
6. Norman AW. Sunlight, season, skin pigmentation, vitamin D, and 25-hydroxyvitamin D: integral components of the vitamin D endocrine system. Am J Clin Nutr. 1998;67(6):1108–10. Oxford University Press.
7. Ponchon G, Kennan A, DeLuca H. "Activation" of vitamin D by the liver. J Clin Invest. 1969;48(11):2032–7.
8. Jetter A, Egli A, Dawson-Hughes B, Staehelin HB, Stoecklin E, Goessl R, et al. Pharmacokinetics of oral vitamin D3 and calcifediol. Bone. 2014;59:14–9.
9. Dusso A, González EA, Martin KJ. Vitamin D in chronic kidney disease. Best Pract Res Clin Endocrinol Metab. 2011;25(4):647–55.
10. Levine B, Singer F, Bryce G, Mallon J, Miller O, Coburn J. Pharmacokinetics and biologic effects of calcitriol in normal humans. J Lab Clin Med. 1985;105(2):234–8.
11. Huang JC, Sakata T, Pfleger LL, Bencsik M, Halloran BP, Bikle DD, et al. PTH differentially regulates expression of RANKL and OPG. J Bone Miner Res. 2004;19(2):235–44.
12. Henry HL. Regulation of vitamin D metabolism. Best Pract Res Clin Endocrinol Metab. 2011;25(4):531–41.
13. Naveh-Many T, Silver J. Regulation of calcitonin gene transcription by vitamin D metabolites in vivo in the rat. J Clin Invest. 1988;81(1):270–3.
14. Pike JW, Meyer MB. The vitamin D receptor: new paradigms for the regulation of gene expression by 1,25-dihydroxyvitamin D(3). Endocrinol Metab Clin N Am. 2010;39(2):255–69.
15. Kongsbak M, Levring T, Geisler C, von Essen M. The vitamin D receptor and T cell function. Front Immunol. 2013;4:148.
16. Xue Y, Fleet JC. Intestinal vitamin D receptor is required for normal calcium and bone metabolism in mice. Gastroenterology. 2009;136(4):1317–27.e2.
17. Johnson JA, Kumar R. Vitamin D and renal calcium transport. Curr Opin Nephrol Hypertens. 1994;3(4):424–9.
18. Kitazawa S, Kajimoto K, Kondo T, Kitazawa R. Vitamin D3 supports osteoclastogenesis via functional vitamin D response element of human RANKL gene promoter. J Cell Biochem. 2003;89(4):771–7.

19. Liu W, Zhang L, Xu H-J, Li Y, Hu C-M, Yang J-Y, et al. The anti-inflammatory effects of vitamin D in tumorigenesis. Int J Mol Sci. 2018;19(9):2736.
20. Ajabshir S, Asif A, Nayer A. The effects of vitamin D on the renin-angiotensin system. J Nephropathol. 2014;3(2):41–3.
21. Al-Badr W, Martin KJ. Vitamin D and kidney disease. Clin J Am Soc Nephrol. 2008;3(5):1555–60.
22. Lips P, van Schoor NM. The effect of vitamin D on bone and osteoporosis. Best Pract Res Clin Endocrinol Metab. 2011;25(4):585–91.
23. Laird E, Ward M, McSorley E, Strain JJ, Wallace J. Vitamin D and bone health: potential mechanisms. Nutrients. 2010;2(7):693–724.
24. Murthy L, Dreyer P, Suriyaarachchi P, Gomez F, Curcio CL, Boersma D, et al. Association between high levels of parathyroid hormone and frailty: the Nepean Osteoporosis and Frailty (NOF) Study. J Frailty Aging. 2018;7(4):253–7.
25. Holick MF. Vitamin D status: measurement, interpretation, and clinical application. Ann Epidemiol. 2009;19(2):73–8.
26. Holick MF, Binkley NC, Bischoff-Ferrari HA, Gordon CM, Hanley DA, Heaney RP, et al. Evaluation, treatment, and prevention of vitamin D deficiency: an Endocrine Society clinical practice guideline. J Clin Endocrinol Metab. 2011;96(7):1911–30.
27. Amrein K, Scherkl M, Hoffmann M, Neuwersch-Sommeregger S, Kostenberger M, Tmava Berisha A, et al. Vitamin D deficiency 2.0: an update on the current status worldwide. Eur J Clin Nutr. 2020; https://doi.org/10.1038/s41430-020-0558-y.
28. Thacher TD, Clarke BL. Vitamin D insufficiency. Mayo Clin Proc. 2011;86(1):50–60.
29. Wei J, Zhu A, Ji JS. A comparison study of vitamin D deficiency among older adults in China and the United States. Sci Rep. 2019;9(1):19713.
30. Cashman KD, Dowling KG, Skrabakova Z, Gonzalez-Gross M, Valtuena J, De Henauw S, et al. Vitamin D deficiency in Europe: pandemic? Am J Clin Nutr. 2016;103(4):1033–44.
31. Laird E, O'Halloran AM, Carey D, Healy M, O'Connor D, Moore P, et al. The prevalence of vitamin D deficiency and the determinants of 25(OH)D concentration in older Irish adults: data from the Irish longitudinal study on ageing (TILDA). J Gerontol A Biol Sci Med Sci. 2018;73(4):519–25.
32. Lee MJ, Hsu HJ, Wu IW, Sun CY, Ting MK, Lee CC. Vitamin D deficiency in northern Taiwan: a community-based cohort study. BMC Public Health. 2019;19(1):337.
33. Kim J, Lee Y, Won CW, Kye S, Shim JS. Association of serum vitamin D with frailty in older Korean adults. Maturitas. 2020;134:15–20.
34. Shardell M, Hicks GE, Miller RR, Kritchevsky S, Andersen D, Bandinelli S, et al. Association of low vitamin D levels with the frailty syndrome in men and women. J Gerontol A Biol Sci Med Sci. 2009;64(1):69–75.
35. Buchebner D, Bartosch P, Malmgren L, McGuigan FE, Gerdhem P, Akesson KE. Association between vitamin D, frailty, and progression of frailty in community-dwelling older women. J Clin Endocrinol Metab. 2019;104(12):6139–47.
36. Sousa-Santos AR, Afonso C, Santos A, Borges N, Moreira P, Padrao P, et al. The association between 25(OH)D levels, frailty status and obesity indices in older adults. PLoS One. 2018;13(8):e0198650.
37. Buckinx F, Rolland Y, Reginster JY, Ricour C, Petermans J, Bruyere O. Burden of frailty in the elderly population: perspectives for a public health challenge. Arch Public Health. 2015;73(1):19.
38. Feng Z, Lugtenberg M, Franse C, Fang X, Hu S, Jin C, et al. Risk factors and protective factors associated with incident or increase of frailty among community-dwelling older adults: a systematic review of longitudinal studies. PLoS One. 2017;12(6):e0178383.
39. Hill TR, Aspray TJ. The role of vitamin D in maintaining bone health in older people. Ther Adv Musculoskelet Dis. 2017;9(4):89–95.
40. Kuchuk NO, Pluijm SM, van Schoor NM, Looman CW, Smit JH, Lips P. Relationships of serum 25-hydroxyvitamin D to bone mineral density and serum parathyroid hormone and markers of bone turnover in older persons. J Clin Endocrinol Metab. 2009;94(4):1244–50.

41. Van Schoor NM, Heymans MW, Lips P. Vitamin D status in relation to physical performance, falls and fractures in the Longitudinal Aging Study Amsterdam: a reanalysis of previous findings using standardized serum 25-hydroxyvitamin D values. J Steroid Biochem Mol Biol. 2018;177:255–60.
42. Yoshimura N, Muraki S, Oka H, Iidaka T, Kodama R, Horii C, et al. Do sarcopenia and/or osteoporosis increase the risk of frailty? A 4-year observation of the second and third ROAD study surveys. Osteoporos Int. 2018;29(10):2181–90.
43. Houston DK, Cesari M, Ferrucci L, Cherubini A, Maggio D, Bartali B, et al. Association between vitamin D status and physical performance: the InCHIANTI study. J Gerontol A Biol Sci Med Sci. 2007;62(4):440–6.
44. Aspell N, Laird E, Healy M, Lawlor B, O'Sullivan M. Vitamin D deficiency is associated with impaired muscle strength and physical performance in community-dwelling older adults: findings from the English longitudinal study of ageing. Clin Interv Aging. 2019;14:1751–61.
45. Wicherts IS, van Schoor NM, Boeke AJ, Visser M, Deeg DJ, Smit J, et al. Vitamin D status predicts physical performance and its decline in older persons. J Clin Endocrinol Metab. 2007;92(6):2058–65.
46. Fritz S, Lusardi M. White paper: "walking speed: the sixth vital sign". J Geriatr Phys Ther. 2009;32(2):46–9.
47. Annweiler C, Henni S, Walrand S, Montero-Odasso M, Duque G, Duval GT. Vitamin D and walking speed in older adults: systematic review and meta-analysis. Maturitas. 2017;106:8–25.
48. Boersma D, Demontiero O, Mohtasham Amiri Z, Hassan S, Suarez H, Geisinger D, et al. Vitamin D status in relation to postural stability in the elderly. J Nutr Health Aging. 2012;16(3):270–5.
49. Akdeniz S, Hepguler S, Ozturk C, Atamaz FC. The relation between vitamin D and postural balance according to clinical tests and tetrax posturography. J Phys Ther Sci. 2016;28(4):1272–7.
50. Tieland M, Brouwer-Brolsma EM, Nienaber-Rousseau C, van Loon LJ, De Groot LC. Low vitamin D status is associated with reduced muscle mass and impaired physical performance in frail elderly people. Eur J Clin Nutr. 2013;67(10):1050–5.
51. Cruz-Jentoft AJ, Bahat G, Bauer J, Boirie Y, Bruyere O, Cederholm T, et al. Sarcopenia: revised European consensus on definition and diagnosis. Age Ageing. 2019;48(1):16–31.
52. Yeung SSY, Reijnierse EM, Pham VK, Trappenburg MC, Lim WK, Meskers CGM, et al. Sarcopenia and its association with falls and fractures in older adults: a systematic review and meta-analysis. J Cachexia Sarcopenia Muscle. 2019;10(3):485–500.
53. Cesari M, Landi F, Vellas B, Bernabei R, Marzetti E. Sarcopenia and physical frailty: two sides of the same coin. Front Aging Neurosci. 2014;6:192.
54. Llewellyn DJ, Lang IA, Langa KM, Melzer D. Vitamin D and cognitive impairment in the elderly U.S. population. J Gerontol A Biol Sci Med Sci. 2011;66(1):59–65.
55. Balion C, Griffith LE, Strifler L, Henderson M, Patterson C, Heckman G, et al. Vitamin D, cognition, and dementia: a systematic review and meta-analysis. Neurology. 2012;79(13):1397–405.
56. Moon JH, Lim S, Han JW, Kim KM, Choi SH, Kim KW, et al. Serum 25-hydroxyvitamin D level and the risk of mild cognitive impairment and dementia: the Korean Longitudinal Study on Health and Aging (KLoSHA). Clin Endocrinol. 2015;83(1):36–42.
57. Lee DH, Chon J, Kim Y, Seo YK, Park EJ, Won CW, et al. Association between vitamin D deficiency and cognitive function in the elderly Korean population: a Korean frailty and aging cohort study. Medicine (Baltimore). 2020;99(8):e19293.
58. Ju SY, Lee JY, Kim DH. Low 25-hydroxyvitamin D levels and the risk of frailty syndrome: a systematic review and dose-response meta-analysis. BMC Geriatr. 2018;18(1):206.
59. Bolzetta F, Veronese N, Stubbs B, Noale M, Vaona A, Demurtas J, et al. The relationship between dietary vitamin K and depressive symptoms in late adulthood: a cross-sectional analysis from a large cohort study. Nutrients. 2019;11(4):787.
60. Muir SW, Montero-Odasso M. Effect of vitamin D supplementation on muscle strength, gait and balance in older adults: a systematic review and meta-analysis. J Am Geriatr Soc. 2011;59(12):2291–300.

61. Stockton KA, Mengersen K, Paratz JD, Kandiah D, Bennell KL. Effect of vitamin D supplementation on muscle strength: a systematic review and meta-analysis. Osteoporos Int. 2011;22(3):859–71.
62. Antoniak AE, Greig CA. The effect of combined resistance exercise training and vitamin D3 supplementation on musculoskeletal health and function in older adults: a systematic review and meta-analysis. BMJ Open. 2017;7(7):e014619.
63. Verlaan S, Maier AB, Bauer JM, Bautmans I, Brandt K, Donini LM, et al. Sufficient levels of 25-hydroxyvitamin D and protein intake required to increase muscle mass in sarcopenic older adults – the PROVIDE study. Clin Nutr. 2018;37(2):551–7.
64. Gillespie LD, Robertson MC, Gillespie WJ, Sherrington C, Gates S, Clemson LM, et al. Interventions for preventing falls in older people living in the community. Cochrane Database Syst Rev. 2012;(9):CD007146.
65. Bischoff-Ferrari HA, Dawson-Hughes B, Staehelin HB, Orav JE, Stuck AE, Theiler R, et al. Fall prevention with supplemental and active forms of vitamin D: a meta-analysis of randomised controlled trials. BMJ. 2009;339:b3692.
66. Kahwati LC, Weber RP, Pan H, Gourlay M, LeBlanc E, Coker-Schwimmer M, et al. Vitamin D, calcium, or combined supplementation for the primary prevention of fractures in community-dwelling adults: evidence report and systematic review for the US Preventive Services Task Force. JAMA. 2018;319(15):1600–12.
67. Bischoff-Ferrari HA, Willett WC, Wong JB, Giovannucci E, Dietrich T, Dawson-Hughes B. Fracture prevention with vitamin D supplementation: a meta-analysis of randomized controlled trials. JAMA. 2005;293(18):2257–64.
68. Sanders KM, Stuart AL, Williamson EJ, Simpson JA, Kotowicz MA, Young D, et al. Annual high-dose oral vitamin D and falls and fractures in older women: a randomized controlled trial. JAMA. 2010;303(18):1815–22.

Chapter 9
Interactions Between "Giants": The Relationship Between Internal Milieu Disorders and Frailty Syndrome

Guido M. Musso-Enz, Olivia M. Capalbo, Henry González-Torres, Gustavo Aroca-Martinez, and Carlos G. Musso

Geriatrics has classically described four entities of its own, naming them "geriatric syndromes" because of their high prevalence and great impact on the senile health. These four significant syndromes, which are more frequently found in older individuals, are delirium, gait disorders and falls, immobility syndrome, and incontinence (urinary and/or fecal). These are all also known as the "geriatric giants," due to their preponderance among older patients and how aggressive they are for their overall health. They can appear as a new acute event (e.g., a previously inexistent gait disorder), or as an exacerbation of an already existing syndrome (e.g., worsening of a previously existent gait disorder). Moreover, these syndromes can often be the only clinical expression of various diseases such as pneumonia, urinary infection, cardiac infarction, etc. In this sense, these diseases can be paucisymptomatic in older people and hence are usually diagnosed thanks to the detection of the

G. M. Musso-Enz
Facultad de Medicina, Universidad Católica Argentina, Buenos Aires, Argentina

O. M. Capalbo
Physiology Department, Instituto Universitario de Buenos Aires, Buenos Aires, Argentina

H. González-Torres
Facultad de Ciencias de la Salud, Universidad Simon Bolivar, Barranquilla, Colombia

Universidad del Valle, Cali, Colombia

G. Aroca-Martinez
Facultad de Ciencias de la Salud, Universidad Simon Bolivar, Barranquilla, Colombia

Nephrology Division, Clinica de la Costa, Barranquilla, Colombia

C. G. Musso (✉)
Nephrology Division, Hospital Italiano de Buenos Aires, Buenos Aires, Argentina

Ageing Biology Unit, Hospital Italiano de Buenos Aires, Buenos Aires, Argentina

Physiology Department, Instituto Universitario del Hospital Italiano de Buenos Aires, Buenos Aires, Argentina
e-mail: carlos.musso@hospitalitaliano.org.ar

© Springer Nature Switzerland AG 2021

C. G. Musso et al. (eds.), *Frailty and Kidney Disease*,
https://doi.org/10.1007/978-3-030-53529-2_9

geriatric giants. If pneumonia or urinary infection appears in young people, they would suffer from symptoms such as cough, fever, dysuria, etc., which in older patients would not commonly appear. This situation has led to the misconception that illnesses in older individuals are oligosyntomatic when in fact their symptomatology is a very rich one, but different respect to the one observed in younger people. Their symptoms are precisely the geriatric giants [1].

Delirium

Delirium is one of the two entities which are directly related with confusional states in older adults, together with dementia. Delirium involves a disturbance of consciousness with impaired alertness and attention. These symptoms could be presented as lethargy or decreased arousability, although intermittent periods of agitation can also occur. On the other hand, patients who suffer from dementia are consistently arousable, as well as capable of staying focused and alert without any effect on their consciousness level. Dementia usually begins and gradually increases, at a very slow rate. Changes only become detectable after long period, generally over weeks, months, and even years. In contrast, delirium undergoes quicker progressions, and develops under a short amount of time, becoming evident over a few minutes, hours, or days. Delirium can be induced by many medical conditions, such as internal milieu disturbances, cerebral hypoperfusion, infections, polypharmacy, etc. It is difficult to identify a single cause of delirium since usually various factors are considered to cause or contribute to aggravate the confusion. It is worth mentioning that not the whole population is prone to developing delirium, but there are risk factors which increase the chances, such as an age older than 65 years, preexistent brain damage, or sensory loss. Some interventions are recommended to be applied in order to reduce confusion, like setting a calendar and a clock in the patient's vision range, constantly promoting conversations, and surrounding the patient with personal possessions (pictures, home decorations, etc.), increase sensory stimulation, and respect patient's sleep-wake cycles [2, 3].

Gait Disorders and Falls

Gait disorders and falls are among the most recurrent clinical complications in older people, being the sixth leading cause of death in this population. These disorders provoke incidents such as fractures (mainly pelvis fracture) or soft tissue injuries which are prone to increase patient's morbidity and mortality.

Even though a fall does not necessarily mean that the patient is at risk of suffering repetitive falls, over two falls during a 6-month lapse are considered abnormal, and it is advised that the patient requires to receive an intense evaluation and to be constantly supervised by professionals. Further interventions such as exercise can improve functional status and reduce the risk of falls. Besides, several falls which occur during a specific amount of time can be an indicator of an underlying acute condition (sepsis, etc.), so in these cases an acute illness should be ruled out. Falls have both extrinsic and intrinsic causes which can also be considered as risk factors. The intrinsic factors are aspects which are specific from each individual, such as chronic diseases, age-related physical and mental changes, acute health problems, or acute exacerbation of chronic disease. Sometimes, intrinsic factors are not the direct cause of a fall, but can aggravate a person's mobility, leading to an increase in the individual's tendency to fall. These may be conditions such as arthritis, cardiovascular insufficiency, neuromuscular diseases, stroke, and reduced vision or hearing ability. The extrinsic factors involve any condition independent to the individual, such as a hazardous environment (e.g., unstable furniture, etc.) or activities (laborer, etc.) [2, 4, 5].

Immobility Syndrome

This "giant" constitutes a common problem which is associated to a great number of diseases in the older population, frequently produces functional decline, and increases the risk of nursing home placement and medical complications. Patient's deconditioning is usually induced by excessive bed rest and is an important clinical entity characterized by several complications such as depression, lethargy, anorexia, dehydration, hypernatremia, hypercalcemia neuromuscular instability, osteoporosis, sarcopenia, incoordination, constipation, as well as urinary and fecal incontinence. Moreover, some authors even characterize frailty as a failure of cognition, mobility, or both. Patients who suffer from immobility syndrome should receive an assessment that includes causes and complications of this syndrome in order to plan their rehabilitation [2, 6, 7].

Urinary Incontinence

Urinary incontinence is defined as the involuntary loss of urine, severe enough to cause social or hygienic problems. This condition affects the patient's life in a variety of ways, including social isolation, depression, stress, skin breakdown, recurrent urinary tract infections, falls, and high economic costs. Approximately 15–30% of older people and 50% of institutionalized older individuals suffer from this "giant." It causes great dependency and disability, being extremely hard for both the patient and their family to try to overcome it and live with it.

Urinary incontinence can present as an acute and reversible form, or a persistent one. Acute reversible urinary incontinence has a sudden onset and is usually associated with an acute medical illness or an iatrogenic cause. On the other hand, persistent urinary incontinence occurs over time and is unrelated to acute events. Once a patient suffers from persistent urinary incontinence, different isolated cases of acute reversible incontinence can aggravate and continue to deteriorate persistent incontinence. This syndrome has four basic causes, and each one of these affects the patient in a particular way. They are delirium, restricted mobility, infections, and drugs. Even though urinary incontinence is not part of normal aging, it comes along with aging-related changes in the urinary tract (decreased bladder capacity, increased prostate size, etc.) which do not cause incontinence but can predispose it [2, 8, 9].

The Nephrogeriatric Giants

Serum electrolyte levels are in normal range in healthy older individuals, but they can be easily altered compared to the young individuals. This phenomenon can be attributed to a reduced homeostatic capability which is tightly related with the significant and prevalent changes suffered by the aged kidney, known as the *nephrogeriatric giants*, which are the following ones [1, 10]:

- Age-related glomerular filtration rate reduction at a rate of 1 ml/year since 40 years of age.
- Tubular dysfunction which consists of reduced sodium reabsorption capability in thick ascending limb of loop of Henle and collecting tubules, reduced water reabsorption capability in collecting tubules, reduced potassium secretion capability in collecting tubules, and reduced free water clearance in thick ascending limb of loop of Henle.
- Medulla hypotonicity, which contributes to the urine concentration capability reduction usually documented in older individuals. Antidiuretic hormone release is not impaired with aging, but this hormone level is relatively increased in older subjects for any given plasma osmolality level compared to the young, indicating a sort of vasopressin kidney resistance.

Interactions Between the "Giants"

It is worth pointing out that the geriatric syndromes (geriatric giants) and the aging-related renal functional changes (nephrogeriatric giants) are clinical entities characteristic in older subjects that predispose to one another and potentiate each other, leading to internal milieu disorders and catastrophic clinical events [11].

For instance, if an older man suffers from urinary infection and because of that he develops delirium (geriatric giant), his feverish state leads him to lose water and also reduces his water intake because of his confusion. Since older individuals have their water reabsorption capability reduced (nephrogeriatric giant), he develops severe dehydration and hypernatremia that worsens his confusional status giving place to a catastrophic clinical event. This clinical case represents an example of a geriatric giant (delirium) that is worsened by a nephrogeriatric giant (reduced water reabsorption capacity) [11, 12] (Fig. 9.1).

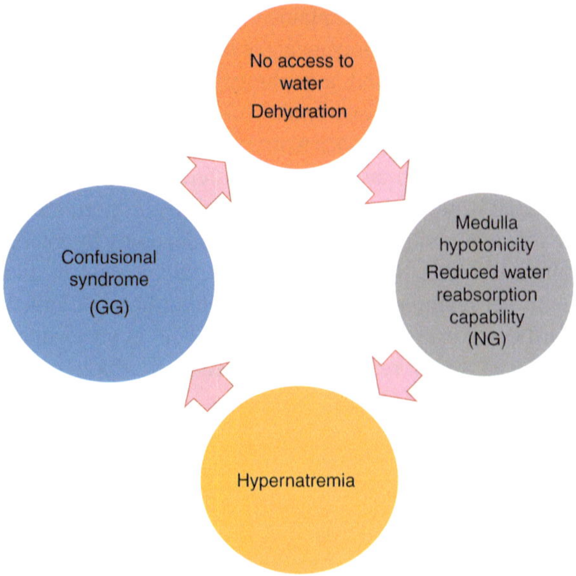

Fig. 9.1 Interdependence between geriatric giant (GG) and nephrogeriatric giant (NG)

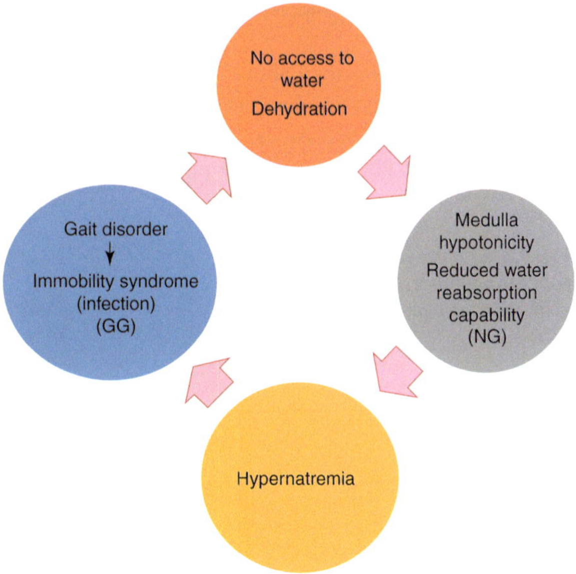

Fig. 9.2 Interdependence between geriatric giant (GG) and nephrogeriatric giant (NG)

Another example could be the case of an older man who lives alone and suffers from gait disorders (geriatric giant) and worsens his condition to immobility syndrome because of an acute respiratory infection. This situation impedes his access to water and consequently leads him to dehydration. Moreover, his reduced water reabsorption capability secondary to his aged kidney (nephrogeriatric giant) contributes to aggravate this dehydration, which in turn worsens his immobility syndrome, leading to a further water depletion (Fig. 9.2).

These previously explained two clinical cases are examples of how a nephrogeriatric giant can aggravate a geriatric giant [11, 12].

On the other hand, a nephrogeriatric giant can be worsened by a geriatric giant leading also to a catastrophic clinical event.

For instance, an older woman who is under the effect of a very hot weather loses water (sweating), and she also suffers from primary hypodipsia and has a reduced salt and water reabsorption capacity (nephrogeriatric giant), both induced by aging-associated changes. Therefore, she develops hypotension which causes dizziness, alters her gait, and finally induces falls (geriatric giant). This situation interferes with her adequate nutrition, worsening her salt and water intake leading her to a further severe volume contraction. This is an example of a nephrogeriatric giant (reduced water reabsorption capability) which is worsened by a geriatric giant (falls) (Fig. 9.3) [10, 11].

Another example of a nephrogeriatric giant which is aggravated by a geriatric giant could be a clinical case of an older man who starts taking an angiotensin II receptor blocker, and since he has a reduced potassium secretion capability due to his aged kidney (nephrogeriatric giant), he develops hyperkalemia. This hyperkalemia induces his a bradyarrhythmia which reduces his cardiac output leading him to cerebral hypoperfusion and confusion (geriatric giant). In this context, he develops dehydration, renal hypoperfusion, renal failure, and more potassium retention (Fig. 9.4) [10, 13].

All the cases described above are examples of what is named as the "feedback between geriatric syndromes." The roots of this phenomenon are in the aging process, because the latter consists of a loss of complexity. An organism (macrosystem) is a system that is constituted by other smaller ones (cardiovascular, respiratory,

Fig. 9.3 Interdependence between nephrogeriatric giant (NG) and geriatric giant (GG)

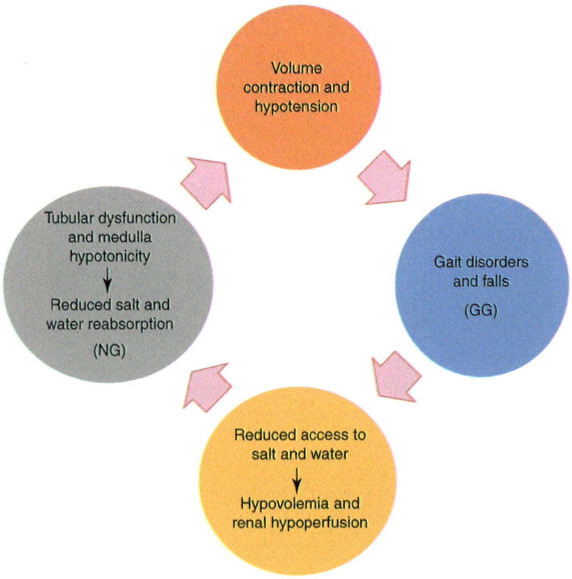

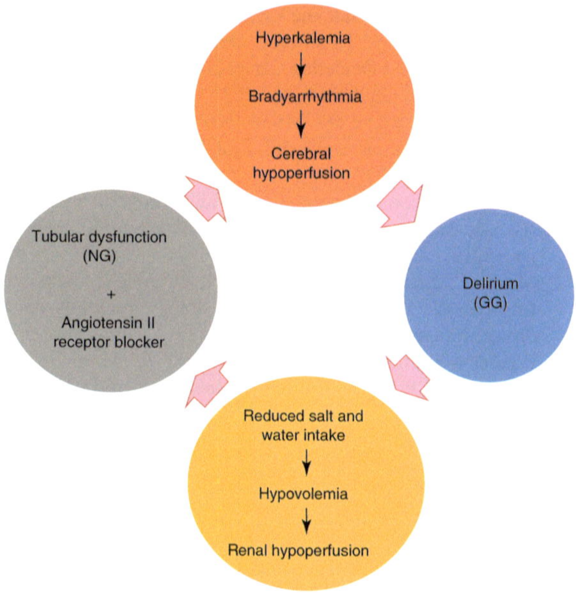

Fig. 9.4 Interdependence between nephrogeriatric giant (NG) and geriatric giant (GG)

etc.) known as microsystems. Complexity means all these microsystems are working harmoniously. An organism functions due to coordination among their multiple microsystems, and this coordination or complexity makes the organism flexible and capable to overcome environmental changes. Aging weakens these microsystems and coordination between them, undermining complexity and making older people frail. Older individuals function normally under basal conditions, but they cannot handle extreme environmental changes, and therefore an otherwise simple event (e.g., hot climate) can lead them to severe compromise or death [11].

Conclusion

Geriatric syndromes (geriatric giant) and the aging-related renal functional changes (nephrogeriatric giants) characteristically predispose and potentiate each other, leading to a vicious cycle of internal milieu disorders and catastrophic clinical events.

References

1. Musso CG. Geriatric nephrology and the "nephrogeriatric giants". Int Urol Nephrol. 2002;34(2):255–6.
2. Forciea M, Lavizzo-Mourey R, Schwab E. Geriatric secrets. Philaelphia: Hanley & Belfus; 2000.

3. National Clinical Guideline Centre for Acute and Chronic Conditions; National Institute for Health and Clinical Excellence. Delirium: prevention, diagnosis and management. London: National Clinical Guideline Centre/National Institute for Health and Care Excellence; 2010. (NICE Clinical Guidelines, No. 103.)
4. Musso CG, Jauregui JR, Macías Núñez JF. Frailty phenotype and chronic kidney disease: a review of the literature. Int Urol Nephrol. 2015;47(11):1801–7. https://doi.org/10.1007/s11255-015-1112-z.
5. Montero-Odasso M, Speechley M. Falls in cognitively impaired older adults: implications for risk assessment and prevention. J Am Geriatr Soc. 2018;66(2):367–75. https://doi.org/10.1111/jgs.15219.
6. Musso C, Liakopoulos V, Pangre N, DiTrolio J, Jauregui R, De Miguel R, Stefanidis I, Imperiali N, Algranati L. Renal physiology in elderly persons with severe immobility syndrome. Int Urol Nephrol. 2009;41(2):437–41. https://doi.org/10.1007/s11255-009-9551-z.
7. Clerencia-Sierra M, Calderón-Larrañaga A, Martínez-Velilla N, Vergara-Mitxeltorena I, Aldaz-Herce P, Poblador-Plou B, Machón-Sobrado M, Egüés-Olazabal N, Abellán-van Kan G, Prados-Torres A. Multimorbidity patterns in hospitalized older patients: associations among chronic diseases and geriatric syndromes. PLoS One. 2015;10(7):e0132909. https://doi.org/10.1371/journal.pone.0132909. eCollection 2015.
8. Searcy JAR. Geriatric urinary incontinence. Nurs Clin North Am. 2017;52(3):447–55. https://doi.org/10.1016/j.cnur.2017.04.002.
9. Musso CG, Alvarez-Gregori J, Jauregui J, Núñez JF. Are currently GFR estimating equations and standard Kt/V value adequate for advanced chronic kidney disease (CKD) frail elderly patients? Int Urol Nephrol. 2015;47(7):1231–2. https://doi.org/10.1007/s11255-015-1010-4.
10. Musso CG, Alvarez Gregori J, Jauregui JR, Macías Núñez JF. Creatinine, urea, uric acid, water and electrolytes renal handling in the healthy oldest old. World J Nephrol. 2012;1(5):123–6. https://doi.org/10.5527/wjn.v1.i5.123.
11. Musso CG, Núñez JF. Feed-back between geriatric syndromes: general system theory in geriatrics. Int Urol Nephrol. 2006;38(3–4):785–6.
12. Turgutalp K, Özhan O, Gök Oğuz E, Yılmaz A, Horoz M, Helvacı I, Kiykim A. Community-acquired hypernatremia in elderly and very elderly patients admitted to the hospital: clinical characteristics and outcomes. Med Sci Monit. 2012;18(12):CR729–34.
13. Lacy C, Armstrong L, Goldman M, Lance L. Drug information handbook. Hudson: Lexi-Comp; 2004.

Chapter 10
Frailty in Acute Kidney Injury Critical Care Patient

María Eugenia González, Nora Angélica Fuentes, Carlos Lautaro Franco, Mateo Lombardi, Carlos Guido Musso, and Elbio Mariano Esperatti

AKI and Frailty in Critical Care Patients

Fragility is a term used to describe a condition characterized by the loss of biological reserve and the vulnerability to restore the homeostasis of subjects after a stressful event [1]. It implies a limited capacity to face the physiological alteration that generates an acute illness, and although it becomes more prevalent with age, it is not exclusive of older individuals [2, 3]. Frailty occurs most frequently in older adults and, similar to acute kidney injury (AKI), carries a high risk of poor outcomes such as physical disability, functional decline, frequent hospitalizations, and increased mortality, particularly in critically ill older patients admitted to the intensive care unit (ICU) [4].

AKI occurs in approximately 20% of hospitalized patients, and the incidence doubles in patients admitted to the intensive care units (ICUs). AKI carries high morbidity, resource utilization, and mortality, particularly in critically ill patients in

M. E. González · N. A. Fuentes · E. M. Esperatti (✉)
Hospital Privado de Comunidad, Mar del Plata, Argentina

Escuela Superior de Medicina, Universidad Nacional de Mar del Plata, Mar del Plata, Argentina
e-mail: nora.fuentes@hospitalitaliano.org.ar

C. L. Franco · M. Lombardi
Physiology Department, Instituto Universitario del Hospital Italiano de Buenos Aires, Buenos Aires, Argentina

C. G. Musso
Physiology Department, Instituto Universitario del Hospital Italiano de Buenos Aires, Buenos Aires, Argentina

Ageing Biology Unit, Hospital Italiano de Buenos Aires, Buenos Aires, Argentina

Nephrology Division, Hospital Italiano de Buenos Aires, Buenos Aires, Argentina

Facultad de Ciencias de la Salud, Universidad Simón Bolívar, Barranquilla, Colombia

© Springer Nature Switzerland AG 2021

C. G. Musso et al. (eds.), *Frailty and Kidney Disease*,
https://doi.org/10.1007/978-3-030-53529-2_10

whom mortality rates could be as high as 50% [5]. Survivors of AKI are susceptible to kidney- and non-kidney-related complications such as the development or progression of chronic kidney disease (CKD), end-stage renal disease (ESRD), and cardiovascular disease. Moreover, survivors of AKI are also at higher risk of early rehospitalization and increased risk of long-term mortality [6].

The incidence of AKI and severe AKI (requiring dialysis) has been increasing over the past decade, and a significant factor contributing to this increase is the old age of population, which is considered an independent risk factor for AKI. Furthermore, elderly patients with AKI have worse renal recovery rate and higher mortality rate than younger patients with AKI [7]. Despite frailty and AKI being commonly encountered in critically ill and older patients, their interplay and interaction remain unclear. Nonetheless, it is possible that they predispose to each other in a vicious circle and therefore worsen patient's overall prognosis [4].

Two recent studies explore the association between AKI and frailty. In one, more than half of the survivors of critical illness who experienced AKI were frail 3 and 12 months after hospital discharge. Further, AKI was associated with worse clinical frailty scores in survivors after adjusting for illness severity. This relationship was robust for severe AKI (KDIGO stages 3) and appeared stronger if injury persisted to hospital discharge. It appears that the severity of AKI and persistence of AKI at discharge from the hospital provided the most striking associations with frailty [3]. On the other hand, frailty was a predictor for the development of AKI in older patietns inpatients. Clinical outcomes, including the likelihood of discharge to nursing facility and short-term and long-term all-cause mortality, were associated with frailty, independent of the severity of AKI [7].

Both studies were conducted in only one center, with a small number of patients, with which the results have little external validity (generalization). Moreover, the fragility and AKI assessment methods were also different; therefore, the results may not be comparable. Thus, further investigations are needed to confirm these initial results.

Anyway, these results are not totally surprising. It is well-known that frailty is more frequent in patients who have chronic kidney disease and that multiple metabolic and nutritional abnormalities may contribute to such association. It is possible that overall frailty status correlates with lower renal functional reserve, therefore constituting an independent risk factor for developing AKI. In the same way, complex physiologic derangements were associated with acute renal failure, and the level of care required in AKI contributed at least to a nutritional defect, poor mobility and possibly sarcopenia which are key determinants of frailty, and cross-talk alteration. In addition, some injury patterns of AKI such as inflammation (cytokines including interleukin-6 and tumor necrosis factor-α) and immune system dysregulation may predispose to frailty. Therefore, frail patients might be vulnerable to AKI through the same inflammatory response. Further, some AKI consequences such as

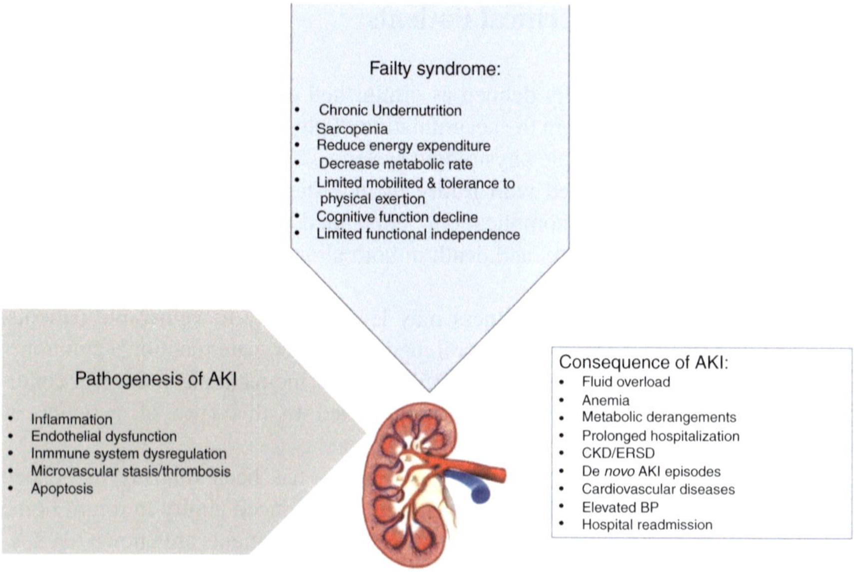

Fig. 10.1 Overview of the potential interplay between frailty and acute kidney injury (AKI)

fluid overload, anemia, cardiovascular disease, and metabolic derangements may also affect the frailty status of some susceptible critical illness survivors [4, 8]. See Figure 10.1.

Other factors that may be present in fragile patients (e.g., polypharmacy, etc.) are associated with an increased risk of AKI in the older individual. There are also treatments that may be indicated in frailty, such as vitamin D. Its overdose is also associated with AKI [9]. On the other hand, frail patients have decreased physiological renal reserve. In fact, one of the studies mentioned previously frailty directly affects AKI incidence and is an independent risk factor for the development of AKI [7].

For critical care providers, these findings highlight that critical illness survivors with AKI, especially those with severe or persistent injury, are at higher risk for clinical frailty for a prolonged duration. Interventions such as physical rehabilitation (including home-based therapy), nutritional evaluation and supplementation (and home-based meal assistance if necessary), and psychosocial support (including psychiatric evaluation and efforts to increase social engagement) may improve or mitigate the development of frailty. Hence, close attention to these factors is necessary, especially during transitions of care. Further, these findings may inform patients and their families regarding the increased probability for a prolonged rehabilitation and for experiencing important patient-centered manifestations of clinical frailty, such as fatigue, slowing, and decrements in independence [3].

Outcomes in Frailty Critical Patients

Frailty has been conceptually defined as diminished physiological reserve associated with age that results from the accumulation of physiologic stresses and comorbid diseases affecting multiple physiologic systems [10, 11].

Adverse events associated with frailty include incident falls, susceptibility to acute illness, perioperative complications, unplanned hospital admissions, disability, need for institutional care, and death in both clinical and surgical care settings [12–14].

The development of critical illness may lead to frailty in vulnerable patients. Critical illness may also be a key factor impeding recovery and functional autonomy in those already considered to be frail [15], both for the pathophysiological conditions and for those linked to the care provided to this type of patients, as described below.

Across multiple measurement strategies, frailty has been robustly associated with worse in-hospital and long-term mortality and reduced ability to return home for both acutely and critically ill patients [16–19]. Frail patients are known to experience poor results in terms of long-term outcomes. Nevertheless, it is less known about how frailty manifests itself in patients' physiology during critical illness and how it affects resource use in intensive care units (ICUs), everything referring to short-term outcomes and organ support used by critically ill patients. In a large cohort of critically ill patients, belonging to 93 ICUs in Brazil, using the modified frailty index (MFI), they founded that frailty was associated not only with in-hospital mortality but also with higher need for organ support during ICU stay (mechanical ventilation, noninvasive ventilation, renal replacement therapy, requirement of vasopressors and blood transfusions), lower probability of returning home with no need for nursing assistance, and longer ICU and hospital length of stay. In addition, there was a dose-response relationship in the MFI results and all its outcomes. MFI values ≥ 3 could be more robust to identify fragility in critical patients, according to these results [20].

Frailty is independently associated with short-term outcomes and resource use in critically ill patients. This has important implications for both administrators and clinicians. Increasing resource use by growing numbers of frail patients must be anticipated. Moreover, their worse prognosis compared to robust patients must be accurately communicated to families and incorporated into decision-making. Because a large number of fragile patients receive critical care and have higher mortality, it would be appropriate to think specialized care for them. For this, further research would be required to provide us with evidence in this scenario [18, 20]. Such programs could have elements that address the minimization of unnecessary sedation [21], detection of delirium [22], early evaluation for weaning of mechanical ventilation, nutritional support [23], medication reconciliation [24], and early mobilization [25, 26]. All these recommended measures in critical patients would be of vital importance in this subpopulation.

In addition, the measurement and diagnosis of frailty could translate into better informed decision-making for patients, their families, and clinicians around issues related to the provision of advanced life support and designation of goals of care. Fragility is a common state that precedes death. Two-thirds of fragile patients have disabling trajectories at the end of life [27]. In a recent population-based study, 26.7% of deaths were associated with frailty. In addition, fragility was associated with high utilization of health services, with most of the expenses related to long-term care and end-of-life hospital care. In fact, health expenses for fragile people increase 2.4 times on average in the last 3 months of life [28].

Tools to Evaluate Frailty in Critical Patients

Several clinical tools have been developed to help in the diagnosis of the frailty syndrome. The most commonly used are (I) the physical frailty phenotype (PFP), which identifies frailty phenotypes based on the examination of changes in weight, weakness, and walking speed; (II) the comprehensive geriatric assessment (CGA), which examines medical, psychosocial, and functional limitations of older adults by a multidisciplinary team of healthcare professionals with the objective of creating a treatment plan of long-term support and rehabilitation for frail adults; and (III) the Clinical Frailty Scale (CFS), which uses pictographs to subjectively stratify older adults according to their level of vulnerability to have poor outcomes such as prolonged hospitalizations and increased mortality. Several studies have attempted to validate and compare these tools, but none of the tools have shown to be superior to their counterparts, and therefore there is no single tool for assessment of frailty postulated as standard of care [4, 29, 30].

There is a wide range of methods to assess the fragility in the literature, whose usefulness depends on the purpose, the environment, the time available, and the ability of the evaluator [31]. The validity and reliability of an evaluation tool is largely dependent on the context and the population in which it has been developed and validated [32]. The assessment of fragility in critical illness leads to particular challenges. Pugh and colleagues in their review conclude that there is little evidence of reliability and only limited evidence on the feasibility of assessing frailty in critically ill patients. The Clinical Frailty Scale (CFS) was the most widely applied evaluation tool by physicians, the conventional evaluation of the physical frailty phenotype (PFP) required modifications for the general application in critical care settings, and the evaluation based on the Fragility Index (FI) may be difficult to perform by the critical care team routinely [2]. Despite a moderate to substantial level of agreement when CFS scores were made binary to distinguish frail from non-frail, there is a statistically and clinically significant discordance between surrogates' and researchers' CFS scores, with surrogates identifying fewer patients as frail than researchers did. This discordance occurred even though surrogates provided most of the baseline demographic and medical information that study investigators used to inform their frailty assessments. In addition, surrogates' and researchers' frailty assessments appeared to differ with respect to the adverse hospital outcomes of mortality, prolonged hospital stay, and incident disability at hospital discharge; investigators were more likely to identify frailty in patients with adverse hospital outcomes. These results have potential research and clinical implications [33].

Scoring systems to stratify risk are a key part of decision-making in modern medicine. In the critical care setting, the most commonly used Acute Physiology and Chronic Health Evaluation II (APACHE-II) score [34] predicts hospital mortality based on acute physiological measurements, age, and a select few severe comorbidities. Frailty scoring quantifies functional reserve, dependence, and vulnerability [14, 35]. Frailty has been shown to predict risk of death better than measures of comorbidity [35] and age alone [16, 36, 37]. Furthermore, acute physiology scores can have significant error especially in the longer term [38, 39]. Incorporating measures of fragility in severity scores could improve the predictive performance of the scores currently used, such as APACHE-II. Since these do not consider key factors of general health that affect mortality, facilitate more informed decision-making in ICU, or prior to critical illness, for issues such as giving more adequate information for decision-making in the ICU on issues such as maximum attention limits [40], adequate referral, or the need for early interventions to reverse the fragility trajectory and improve outcomes. However, before the fragility score can be used to influence decision-making in the ICU, its relationship with the results in critical patients must be thoroughly tested [14].

Data from literature suggest that frailty can be measured in patients admitted to the ICU using a simple bedside assessment tool and is an important prognostic factor in both the short and long term [41].

Conclusion

In summary, the study by Abdel-Kader et al. revealed a novel and independent association between AKI and subsequent frailty status at 3 and 12 months in survivors from critical illness. This important observational study could lead to investigate the mechanisms that could link both of these syndromes and how they could potentially predispose to each other. It is possible that the overall patient's frailty status correlates with his/her renal functional reserve and consequently constitutes an independent risk factor for developing AKI. In addition, some injury patterns of AKI such as inflammation and immune system dysregulation may predispose to frailty. Further, some AKI consequences such as fluid overload, anemia, cardiovascular disease, and metabolic derangements may also affect the frailty status of some susceptible critical illness survivors. Further studies should validate these findings, underpin potential mechanisms of this—possibly bidirectional—association, and, importantly, develop therapeutic strategies focused on ameliorating the burden of frailty in survivors of critical illness and AKI.

References

1. Clegg A, Young J, Iliffe S, Rikkert MO, Rockwood K. Frailty in elderly people. Lancet. 2013;381:752–62.
2. Pugh RJ, Ellison A, Pye K, Subbe CP, Thorpe CM, Lone NI, et al. Feasibility and reliability of frailty assessment in the critically ill: a systematic review. Crit Care. 2018;22(1):49. https://doi.org/10.1186/s13054-018-1953-9.
3. Abdel-Kader K, Girard TD, Brummel NE, Saunders CT, Blume JD, Clark AJ, et al. Acute kidney injury and subsequent frailty status in survivors of critical illness: a secondary analysis. Crit Care Med. 2018;46:e380–8.
4. Ortiz-Soriano V, Neyra JA. The impact of acute kidney injury on frailty status in critical illness survivors-is there enough evidence? J Emerg Crit Care Med. 2018;2:93. https://doi.org/10.21037/jeccm.2018.10.17.
5. Rewa O, Bagshaw SM. Acute kidney injury-epidemiology, outcomes and economics. Nat Rev Nephrol. 2014;10:193–207.
6. Li PKT, Burdmann EA, Mehta RL. World Kidney Day 2013: acute kidney injury-global health alert. Am J Kidney Dis. 2013;61:359–63.
7. Baek SH, Lee SW, Kim S-W, Ahn SY, Yu M-Y, Kim K-I, et al. Frailty as a predictor of acute kidney injury in hospitalized elderly patients: a single center, retrospective cohort study. PLoS One. 2016;11:e0156444.
8. Arnouat M, Launey Y, Seguin P. Acute kidney injury in critical illness and long-term frailty: a new challenge for intensivists? J Emerg Crit Care Med. 2018;2:4. https://doi.org/10.21037/jeccm.2018.10.01.
9. Chowdry AM, Azad H, Najar MS, Mir I. Acute kidney injury due to overcorrection of hypovitaminosis D: a tertiary center experience in the Kashmir Valley of India. Saudi J Kidney Dis Transpl. 2017;28:1321–9.
10. Fried LP, Ferrucci L, Darer J, Williamson JD, Anderson G. Untangling the concepts of disability, frailty, and comorbidity: implications for improved targeting and care. J Gerontol A Biol Sci Med Sci. 2004;59:255–63.
11. Farhat JS, Falvo AJ, Mathilda Horst H, Swartz A, Velanovich V, Patton JH, et al. Are the frail destined to fail?: frailty index as a predictor of surgical morbidity and mortality in the elderly. J Am Coll Surg. 2011;213(3):S65. https://doi.org/10.1016/j.jamcollsurg.2011.06.147.
12. Makary MA, Segev DL, Pronovost PJ, Syin D, Bandeen-Roche K, Patel P, et al. Frailty as a predictor of surgical outcomes in older patients. J Am Coll Surg. 2010;210:901–8.
13. Lee DH, Buth KJ, Martin B-J, Yip AM, Hirsch GM. Frail patients are at increased risk for mortality and prolonged institutional care after cardiac surgery. Circulation. 2010;121:973–8.
14. Rockwood K, Song X, Mitnitski A. Changes in relative fitness and frailty across the adult lifespan: evidence from the Canadian National Population Health Survey. CMAJ. 2011;183:E487–94.
15. McDermid RC, Stelfox HT, Bagshaw SM. Frailty in the critically ill: a novel concept. Crit Care. 2011;15:301.
16. Muscedere J, Waters B, Varambally A, Bagshaw SM, Boyd JG, Maslove D, et al. The impact of frailty on intensive care unit outcomes: a systematic review and meta-analysis. Intensive Care Med. 2017;43:1105–22.
17. Le Maguet P, Roquilly A, Lasocki S, Asehnoune K, Carise E, Saint Martin M, et al. Prevalence and impact of frailty on mortality in elderly ICU patients: a prospective, multicenter, observational study. Intensive Care Med. 2014;40:674–82.
18. Brummel NE, Bell SP, Girard TD, Pandharipande PP, Jackson JC, Morandi A, et al. Frailty and subsequent disability and mortality among patients with critical illness. Am J Respir Crit Care Med. 2017;196:64–72.
19. Ferrante LE, Pisani MA, Murphy TE, Gahbauer EA, Leo-Summers LS, Gill TM. The association of frailty with post-ICU disability, nursing home admission, and mortality: a longitudinal study. Chest. 2018;153:1378–86.

20. Zampieri FG, Iwashyna TJ, Viglianti EM, Taniguchi LU, Viana WN, Costa R, et al. Association of frailty with short-term outcomes, organ support and resource use in critically ill patients. Intensive Care Med. 2018;44:1512–20.
21. Shehabi Y, Chan L, Kadiman S, Alias A, Ismail WN, Tan MATI, et al. Sedation depth and long-term mortality in mechanically ventilated critically ill adults: a prospective longitudinal multicentre cohort study. Intensive Care Med. 2013;39:910–8.
22. Quinlan N, Marcantonio ER, Inouye SK, Gill TM, Kamholz B, Rudolph JL. Vulnerability: the crossroads of frailty and delirium. J Am Geriatr Soc. 2011;59(Suppl 2):S262–8.
23. Doig GS, Simpson F, Finfer S, Delaney A, Davies AR, Mitchell I, et al. Effect of evidence-based feeding guidelines on mortality of critically ill adults: a cluster randomized controlled trial. JAMA. 2008;300:2731–41.
24. Manias E, Williams A, Liew D. Interventions to reduce medication errors in adult intensive care: a systematic review. Br J Clin Pharmacol. 2012;74:411–23.
25. Schweickert WD, Pohlman MC, Pohlman AS, Nigos C, Pawlik AJ, Esbrook CL, et al. Early physical and occupational therapy in mechanically ventilated, critically ill patients: a randomised controlled trial. Lancet. 2009;373:1874–82.
26. Ferrucci L, Guralnik JM, Studenski S, Fried LP, Cutler GB Jr, Walston JD, et al. Designing randomized, controlled trials aimed at preventing or delaying functional decline and disability in frail, older persons: a consensus report. J Am Geriatr Soc. 2004;52:625–34.
27. Gill TM, Gahbauer EA, Han L, Allore HG. Trajectories of disability in the last year of life. N Engl J Med. 2010;362:1173–80.
28. Fassbender K, Fainsinger RL, Carson M, Finegan BA. Cost trajectories at the end of life: the Canadian experience. J Pain Symptom Manag. 2009;38:75–80.
29. Cesari M, Gambassi G, van Kan GA, Vellas B. The frailty phenotype and the frailty index: different instruments for different purposes. Age Ageing. 2014;43:10–2.
30. Aprahamian I, de Castro Cezar NO, Izbicki R, Lin SM, Paulo DLV, Fattori A, et al. Screening for frailty with the FRAIL scale: a comparison with the phenotype criteria. J Am Med Dir Assoc. 2017;18:592–6.
31. Buta BJ, Walston JD, Godino JG, Park M, Kalyani RR, Xue Q-L, et al. Frailty assessment instruments: systematic characterization of the uses and contexts of highly-cited instruments. Ageing Res Rev. 2016;26:53–61.
32. Sutton JL, Gould RL, Daley S, Coulson MC, Ward EV, Butler AM, et al. Psychometric properties of multicomponent tools designed to assess frailty in older adults: a systematic review. BMC Geriatr. 2016;16:55.
33. Hope AA, Munoz M, Hsieh SJ, Gong MN. Surrogates' and researchers' assessments of prehospital frailty in critically ill older adults. Am J Crit Care. 2019;28:117–23.
34. Knaus W, Wagner D, Draper E, Zimmerman J. A physiologic based classification system for critically ill patients. Crit Care Med. 1980;8(4):261. https://doi.org/10.1097/00003246-198004000-00153.
35. Rockwood K, Song X, MacKnight C, Bergman H, Hogan DB, McDowell I, et al. A global clinical measure of fitness and frailty in elderly people. CMAJ. 2005;173:489–95.
36. Bagshaw SM, Majumdar SR, Rolfson DB, Ibrahim Q, McDermid RC, Tom Stelfox H. A prospective multicenter cohort study of frailty in younger critically ill patients. Crit Care. 2016;20(1):175. https://doi.org/10.1186/s13054-016-1338-x.
37. Zeng A, Song X, Dong J, Mitnitski A, Liu J, Guo Z, et al. Mortality in relation to frailty in patients admitted to a specialized geriatric intensive care unit. J Gerontol A Biol Sci Med Sci. 2015;70:1586–94.
38. Baldwin MR, Reid MC, Westlake AA, Rowe JW, Granieri EC, Wunsch H, et al. The feasibility of measuring frailty to predict disability and mortality in older medical intensive care unit survivors. J Crit Care. 2014;29:401–8.
39. Knaus WA, Draper EA, Wagner DP, Zimmerman JE. APACHE II. Crit Care Med. 1985;13(10):818–29. https://doi.org/10.1097/00003246-198510000-00009.

40. de Vries NM, Staal JB, van Ravensberg CD, Hobbelen JSM, Olde Rikkert MGM, Nijhuis-van der Sanden MWG. Outcome instruments to measure frailty: a systematic review. Ageing Res Rev. 2011;10:104–14.
41. Bagshaw SM, Stelfox HT, McDermid RC, Rolfson DB, Tsuyuki RT, Baig N, et al. Association between frailty and short- and long-term outcomes among critically ill patients: a multicentre prospective cohort study. Can Med Assoc J. 2014;186(2):E95–E102. https://doi.org/10.1503/cmaj.130639.

Chapter 11
Frailty in Non-Dialysis Chronic Kidney Disease

Malena Colombo, Victoria P. Musso-Enz, María del Pilar Romero, Gustavo Aroca-Martinez, and Carlos G. Musso

Introduction

Frailty status is a condition which is not merely induced by aging but mainly by a progressive and sustained deterioration of several body physiological processes that lead to an increased vulnerability to stressors [1–7]. The main clinical characteristics of frailty status are low physical activity and poor social connections [5, 8].

The prevalence of frailty and pre-frailty status in older individuals ranges from 7% to 15% and 44% to 47%, respectively. This condition is characteristically more prevalent in women and increases steadily with age from 4% in older individuals (65–69 years) to 26% in the oldest old (≥85 years) [9, 10]. Frailty pathophysiology consists of a simultaneous functional reserve decline (below a 30%) of many systems, such as skeletal muscle, nervous, endocrine, and immune systems, with even poor coordination among their functions, leading to an altered homeostatic response, mediated by metabolic imbalance, cytokine over-expression (TNF-alpha, interleukin-6, interleukin-1), and/or hormonal dysfunction [10, 11].

M. Colombo · V. P. Musso-Enz · M. del P. Romero
Physiology Department, Instituto Universitario del Hospital Italiano de Buenos Aires, Buenos Aires, Argentina

G. Aroca-Martinez
Facultad de Ciencias de la Salud, Universidad Simon Bolivar, Barranquilla, Colombia

C. G. Musso (✉)
Physiology Department, Instituto Universitario del Hospital Italiano de Buenos Aires, Buenos Aires, Argentina

Facultad de Ciencias de la Salud, Universidad Simon Bolivar, Barranquilla, Colombia

Nephrology Division, Hospital Italiano de Buenos Aires, Buenos Aires, Argentina

Ageing Biology Unit, Hospital Italiano de Buenos Aires, Buenos Aires, Argentina
e-mail: carlos.musso@hospitalitaliano.org.ar

© Springer Nature Switzerland AG 2021

C. G. Musso et al. (eds.), *Frailty and Kidney Disease*,
https://doi.org/10.1007/978-3-030-53529-2_11

Frailty status prevalence in non-dialysis chronic kidney disease (CKD) patients is around 14% [10], and CKD associated inflammation, increased oxidative stress, protein-energy wasting, and dysregulated methionine transmethylation reactions contribute to the appearance of frailty in this group [10]. Moreover, some pathological conditions have been suggested as common pathways among frailty and CKD, as is the case of altered hemoglobin, interleukin 6, insulin-like growth factor 1 (IGF-1), dehydroepiandrosterone-S (DHEA-S), hemoglobin A1c (Hb A1c), 25-hydroxy vitamin D, vitamin B12, and, carotenoids levels [5, 7, 12].

This chapter describes the relationship between fragility and CKD, its clinical consequences, and adequate therapeutic approach.

Frailty in Chronic Kidney Disease: Senescent Nephropathy

The prevalence of frailty is higher in older individuals with CKD compared to normal kidney ones, and this prevalence increases with worsening kidney function, having worse outcomes than those that are robust with CKD, including an increased falls, hospitalization, dialysis requirement, and mortality [1, 12]. Frailty phenotype prevalence among end-stage renal disease patients is five- to sevenfold higher than in community-dwelling older adults, and it is linked to higher rates of mortality [9, 11]. The inflammatory state, which characterized both frailty and CKD, is associated with their increase in resting energy expenditure that may contribute to the imbalance of muscle protein homeostasis. The signaling of the anabolic hormones (insulin and IGF-1) is impaired by the proinflammatory cytokines by increasing the glucocorticoids activity, and by directly causing skeletal muscle resistance to insulin and IGF-1. This phenomenon incites muscle protein breakdown via the caspase-3 and ubiquitin proteasome system [12].

According to the Health, Aging and Body Composition Study, an estimated glomerular filtration rate (eGFR) less than 60 ml/min/1.73 m2 was independently associated with the progressive difficulty in walking one-quarter of a mile or climbing a ten-steps stairs. In a follow-up study, participants found in the highest quartile of cystatin C concentration (≥1.13 mg/L) experienced a significantly higher risk of developing functional limitation than those in the lowest quartile (<0.86 mg/L) [13]. The Heart and Soul Study found that exercise capacity was diminished in patients with eGFR <60 ml/min/1.73 m^2 for low exercise capacity, compared to those with eGFR >90 ml/min/1.73 m^2. Further findings demonstrated that maximum exercise tolerance becomes impaired even in early CKD stages, since participants with eGFR 60–90 ml/min/1.73 m^2 were also more likely to have low exercise capacity [13]. It has been documented that stage 3b CKD patients had defective oxygen consumption during maximal exercise, and they also performed poorly on several tests of day-to-day activities, with maximal gait speed over a short distance 85% and sit-to-stand performance 79% of population norms. The proportion of patients who failed to rise from a chair without using their arms was higher among individuals with lower eGFR, and no patients with eGFR <12 ml/min/1.73 m^2 were able to perform this task [13].

Malnutrition is a prevalent condition in end-stage renal disease (ESRD) patients, which gradually progresses with renal function deterioration prior to renal replacement therapy (RRT) initiation. This phenomenon can be induced by reduced dietary intake, uremic toxins accumulation, RRT catabolic effects, oxidative stress, metabolic and hormonal imbalances, increased insulin resistance, systemic inflammation, and comorbid conditions. All these factors can lead to physical, mental, and social deterioration [14].

As mentioned above, CKD predisposes to frailty through many mechanisms, such as anemia, bone fragility, chronic inflammation, oxidative stress, atherosclerosis, malnutrition, sarcopenia, and even all these factors can also lead to CKD progression, giving place to a dangerous vicious cycle. Consequently, CKD in older patients are more likely to reach frailty, and as CKD disease progresses, the prevalence of frailty increases. Meanwhile, frailty status influences negatively CKD evolution as well as the health conditions that chronic nephropathy patients deal with. Therefore, those patients who suffer from CKD and frailty at the same time are at greater risk of falling, showing fractures, getting hospitalized, and they also have more chances of progressing to dialysis and death. Because of that the coexistence of CKD and frailty phenotype has been considered a particular condition named "senescent nephropathy" (SN). SN is characterized by significant clinical complications, therapeutic demands (e.g., rehabilitation), and worse prognosis, in comparison with robust older CKD patients (Table 11.1) [3, 4, 12].

Moreover, a study that compared the worsening of the health-related quality of life (HRQL) in ESRD documented that frailty was associated with worse HRQL at the follow-up, and that it was the only factor that was associated with it. The same study showed that the overall pattern of change in HRQL suggested that most participants had stable HRQL but when there was a change in HRQL, it was more likely to be worse [15]. There is strong evidence that links HRQL with mortality risk in ESRD patients, but not enough studies examined this relationship with earlier stages of CKD [13].

Table 11.1 Differences between chronic kidney disease (CKD) robust older patients and senescent nephropathy (SN) patients

	CKD	SN
CKD diagnosis	Positive	Positive
Frailty score	Negative	Positive
Therapy	Corresponding CKD therapy (conventional tagets)	Corresponding CKD therapy adjusted to frailty status (conventional or modified targets) + Frail rehabilitation & home assistance
Follow-up	Standard control rate	Tighter control rate
Prognosis	Standard	Worse

Sarcopenia and CKD

Sarcopenia, which is defined as musculoskeletal mass and strength reduction, is an important component of the frailty phenotype. Its diagnosis is based on the evaluation of the muscle mass by imaging techniques (computed tomography or magnetic resonance), bioimpedance analysis (lean body mass), muscle strength (handgrip), and the physical performance assessed by applying clinical test, such as the short physical performance battery or timed get-up-and-go test, and/ or applying clinical scores (Table 11.2) [4, 10, 16]. People tend to lose muscle mass at a rate of 1–2% per year after the age of 50 years, due to a progressive atrophy and loss of type II muscle fibers and motor neurons, as well as an increased variability in fiber size, extracellular space expansion, protein aggregates deposition within the interstitial matrix, and increased infiltration of adipose and connective tissues, all changes which contribute to a decline in the muscle functional capability. In addition, other mechanisms involved in the onset and progression of sarcopenia are the low protein diet, reduced growth hormone and androgens serum levels, insulin resistance, low vitamin D, high cortisol levels, metabolic acidosis, and chronic diseases such as diabetes mellitus, cirrhosis, peripheral vascular disease, and CKD [4, 6, 10]. Moreover, muscle loss is more pronounced in pre-dialysis patients, which may ameliorate once dialysis has been initiated [12]. Skeletal muscle biopsies from patients with advanced chronic nephropathy show lower mitochondrial volume density and mitochondrial DNA copy number than controls, changes that can be reversed by muscles resistance exercise [17]. An important contributor to sarcopenia during kidney injury is the skeletal muscle down-regulation by inflammatory mediators such as IL6 and TNF-like weak inducer of apoptosis (TWEAK), being the exercise beneficial effect mediated by TWEAK modulation [14, 17]. Regarding metabolic acidosis, it activates caspase-3 and the ubiquitin proteasome system, inhibiting the intracellular signaling of insulin and IGF-1 and increasing the adrenal glucocorticoid production, resulting in protein catabolism that activate muscle breakdown cytokines (interleukin-6 and TNF-alpha), which finally induce sarcopenia [12, 14]. It is worth mentioning that, social isolation and depression, usually associated to CKD, are also sarcopenia inducing factors since these behaviors lead to inactivity and loss of muscles function [3, 4].

The highest concern of sarcopenia is altered locomotion, but it can also impair other vital functions such as glucose regulation, hormone production, and muscle tissue mass as the major potassium and amino acids body reservoir. Moreover, sarcopenia increases the risk of numerous adverse outcomes such as physical disability, diminished quality of life, and death [10]. In addition, sarcopenia explains why

Table 11.2 Clinical sarcopenia stages

Sarcopenia	Muscle mass	Muscle strength	Performance
Pre-status	Low	Normal	Normal
Mild-moderate	Low	Low	Normal
Severe	Low	Low	Low

when kidney function is assessed in older people using eGFR equations based on serum creatinine, those patients with the lowest and highest eGFR values were associated with the highest mortality (U-shape curve) [10]. This phenomenon is particularly prominent in octogenarians, and probably can be explained by the fact that higher eGFR can reflect those individuals with lower muscle mass and malnutrition [4].

Frailty Evaluation in CKD

Frailty screening should be routinely performed in CKD patients (young or older) so that targeted management strategies can be offered. The two more popular frailty diagnosing tests are: the Fried Frailty Phenotype and the Frailty Index (FI). The former has a more robust evidence base in terms of predicting outcomes in CKD patients, but is a time-consuming evaluation, thus not practical to be performed routinely to nephrology outpatients [1]. Fried et al. created the concept of frailty phenotype that incorporates disturbances across five clinical domains: shrinking, weakness, poor endurance and energy, slowness, and low physical activity level, in order to identify older people who are at risk of disability, falls, institutionalization, hospitalization, and premature death [4, 10]. Those individuals who have ≥3 domains are considered to be frail, those who have one or two altered domains to be vulnerable or pre-frail individuals, and those with no domain to be fit or robust [11]. It is worth pointing out that sarcopenia is usually considered included into the "shrinking" domain; and that social isolation, depression, and cognitive impairment are usually considered as exacerbating conditions of the frailty phenotype [10]. However, as the Fried frailty phenotype was developed in community-dwelling older adults, some components may not be fully applicable to ESRD patients, while there is also some physiological reserve aspect of these patients that are not fully covered by the Fried frailty phenotype [9]. In this sense, since frailty phenotype, comorbidity, and disability are related terms but they should not be used interchangeably, the coexistence of these entities may imply the risk of over-diagnosing frailty phenotype in people whose clinical "domains" are not secondary to their loss of complexity (frailty phenotype) but to their comorbidities (presence of more than three chronic disease) or disability (altered at least one of the daily activities). Thus, to apply Fried frailty score to CKD patients may overreport the true prevalence of frailty in these groups (pseudo-frailty phenotype) [10]. Mitnitski et al. described a holistic approach to assessing frailty in older patient, and Rockwood et al. further developed a frailty diagnostic model, including a total of 70 variables consisting of a variety of medical and psychological conditions and functional impairments. The total number of deficits for an individual patient was divided by all the predetermined clinical variables to calculate in order to obtain a Frailty Index (FI) score. Rockwood et al. then compared the FI with the frailty phenotype, demonstrating that both frailty definitions correlated moderately well with each other. However, FI is hard to implement into routine clinical cares because it requires the assessment of many variables [3, 5, 12]. The Clinical Frailty Scale (CFS) is a frailty screening tool that consists of a 7-point scale with descriptors for levels of frailty that relies on clinical judgement alone, which then it was updated to nine descriptors including two terminality states. Higher scores on the CFS were associated with an increased risk of death and institutionalization. The CFS is the simplest and clinically useful and validated tool for diagnosing frailty, then it seems to be the most recommended test because it integrates known and unrecognized disturbances in multiple organ systems (cardiovascular, respiratory, nervous, and musculoskeletal systems) many of which affect survival [1]. Alfaadhel et al. demonstrated that high CFS scores at dialysis initiation are associated with mortality, and a subsequent study showed that the CFS performed in patient's pre-dialysis is an independent predictor of mortality. In this sense, Iyasere et al. performed the CFS within their study that compared the quality of life and physical function in older patients on assisted peritoneal dialysis and hemodialysis, documenting that higher CFS scores were associated with worse HRQL scores [3, 4, 12] (Table 11.3). Clarke et al. report that the self-reported measures of physical performance Duke Activity Status Index (physical function) and General Practice Physical Activity Questionnaire (habitual activity regarding walking behavior) were independently associated with survival in non-dialysis CKD [17]. Even though self-report responses are simple to complete, they may be confusing or allow respondents to overestimate their capabilities [18]. For instance, from a group of stage 4–5 CKD patients, only 6% self-identified as frail, while in fact,

Table 11.3 Clinical Frailty Scale (CFS) (If dementia is present, the degree of frailty usually corresponds to the degree of dementia)

CFS score	Clinical characteristics
1 - Very fit	People who are robust, active, energetic, and motivated. These people commonly exercise regularly. They are among the fittest for their age.
2 - Well	People who have no active disease symptoms, but are less fit than category 1. Often, they exercise or are very active occasionally.
3 - Managing well	People whose medical problem are well controlled, but are not regularly active beyond routine walking.
4 - Vulnerable	While not dependent on others for daily help, often symptoms limit activities. A common complaint is being "slowed up," and/or being tired during the day.
5 - Mildly frail	These people often have more evident slowing and need help in high orders (finances, medication, transportation, heavy housework).
6 - Moderately frail	People need help with all outdoor activities. Indoors, they need help with housekeeping, and often have problems with stairs. They also need help with bathing and might need minimal assistance with dressing.
7 - Severely frail	Completely dependent for personal care, from either cause (physical or cognitive). Even so, they seem stable and not at high risk of dying.
8 - Very severely frail	Completely dependent, and approaching the end of life (within 6 months).
9 - Terminally ill	Approaching the end of life. This category applies to any people with a life expectancy <6 months, who are not otherwise evidently frail.

20% were measured as frail by applying the Fried phenotype. Besides, it has been documented that among ESRD patients, 91% of whom both measured and self-identified as frail, believed that adults with ESRD just like them are more likely to be frail than healthy adults. However, only 58% of participants who measured as frail but not identified that way believed that adults with ESRD are more likely to be frail [9]. Even though it has been suggested that questionnaire-based frailty assessing methods are more likely to overestimate the patient's capability, they still appear to be predictive of outcomes [12]. Regarding the medical-reports, 98% of clinicians think that adults with ESRD are more likely to be frail than healthy adults. There are three Fried frailty components that at least one clinician identifies as not relevant to adults with ESRD: weight loss, slowed walking, and weak strength. The component most frequently identified as not relevant to adults with ESRD was weight loss, since their weight constantly fluctuates [9]. Regarding frailty diagnostic physical test, the walking speed test showed the highest area under the curve (AUC) value (0.97 [95% CI 0.93–1.00]), but the Frailty Phenotype walking speed criterion cut-off was most discriminative with a sensitivity of 0.84 (95% CI 0.62–0.94) and specificity of 0.96 (95% CI 0.88–0.99). Among the non-physical frailty diagnostic tests, the CFS showed the highest AUC value (0.90 [95% CI 0.84–0.97]). It showed good sensitivity and specificity when using a cut-off of ≥5 (0.79 [95% CI 0.57–0.91] and 0.87 [95% CI 0.78–0.93], respectively [1] (Table 11.1)**.** Finally, Iyasere et al. demonstrated that higher CFS scores are associated with worse HRQL in older patients receiving assisted peritoneal dialysis and hemodialysis. The FI had the worst performance with a low and non-significant AUC value (0.63, 95% CI 0.50–0.78) in CKD. Roshanravan et al. demonstrated that walking speed is associated with mortality in patients with CKD, unlike hand grip strength [1].

It should be taken into account that the low level of physical activity usually found in ESRD patients can tend to over-detect frailty phenotype in this group; then, the reliable tests mentioned above can help to avoid misdiagnose [10].

Senescent Nephropathy Treatment

Frailty status trends should be identified since there is a window of opportunity in which clinicians can successfully intervene by referring patients to interventions aimed at decreasing frailty risk and minimizing premature mortality by optimizing nutritional and rehabilitation [18]. The prevention or delay of the appearance of frailty and sarcopenia can be accomplished mainly by low intensity resistance and aerobic physical exercise, an adequate caloric and protein intake, vitamin D supplementation, and avoidance of polypharmacy. In addition, these patients should also receive their CKD corresponding treatment, but even frailty evaluation can contribute to redesigning patient's therapeutic objectives [16].

There is an increased risk of poor outcomes associated with frailty, leading to the analysis of risk to benefit trade-off of standard treatment options (including renal replacement therapies) for the patient. For instance, nephroprevention objectives for frail CKD older patients should be different from those for robust CKD young patients (Table 11.4) [19]. Therefore, early frailty identification is a vital medical target because of its high and increasing prevalence and to its prognostic importance and influence in the potential medical management (Fig. 11.1) [4].

Table 11.4 Nephroprevention targets (estimative) for chronic kidney disease (CKD) and senescent nephropathy (SN) patients

Nephroprevention targets	CKD conventional targets	SN modified targets (if conventional targets were not tolerated)
Diet	Low sodium Low protein	Normal sodium (to avoid hypotension and/or hyponatremia) Normal protein (to avoid sarcopenia)
Hemoglobin (g/dl)	11	11.5–12 (to avoid cognitive dysfunction and/or falls)
Glycated hemoglobin (HbA_{1C}) (%)	<7	7.5–8.5 (to avoid hypoglycemia)
Blood pressure (mmHg)	≤130–80	≤140/150–80 (to avoid cognitive dysfunction and/or falls) diastolic higher 60 (to avoid coronary event)
Proteinuria (g/day)	<0.5	<1 (to avoid hyperkalemia, hyponatremia, and /or renal function deterioration induced by antiproteinuric drugs)

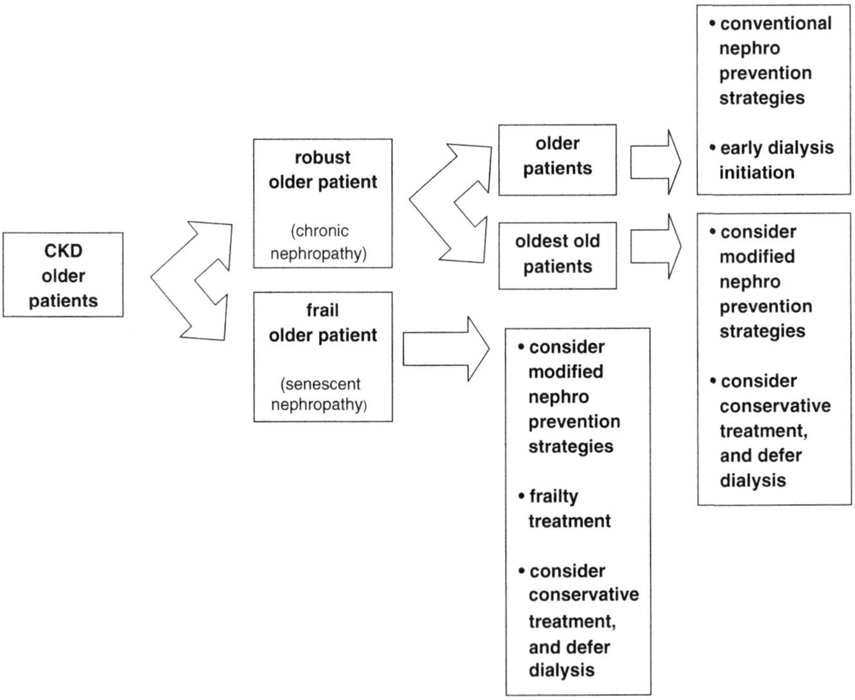

Fig. 11.1 Proposed nephroprevention algorithm in older patients with chronic kidney disease (CKD)

Diet

Patients with advanced CKD often have a reduced energy intake that contributes to sarcopenia and, subsequently, to physical frailty. This is generally due to anorexia which is present in one-third of ESRD patients. This loss of appetite is multifactorial, being its potential contributors the uremic milieu, inflammation, superimposed illnesses, medications, and low mood. Moreover, the uremic toxins accumulation causes defects in the appetite hypothalamic regulation. Cognitive impairment, which is more common in the CKD population, usually leads to reduced food intake. Patients with CKD should maintain an adequate protein and energy intake while restricting dietary phosphate intake to prevent the development of secondary hyperparathyroidism and CKD bone disease [12].

Exercise

Exercise can be used as a treatment for sarcopenia, since its beneficial effect has been associated to improvements in proteolysis, muscle regeneration, and inflammatory cytokines release. Low-intensity resistance and aerobic exercise improved physical fitness, muscular strength, and quality of life not only in ESRD and dialysis patients, but also has positive effects on eGFR and exercise tolerance in stage 3–4 CKD. Unfortunately, limited evidence is available regarding the exercise impact on frailty in earlier stages of CKD [9, 10, 17]. The importance of regular exercise in CKD older patients lies in building up or maintaining their functional capacity and independence [5]. In this sense, an exercise counseling clinic could be an option to prevent the progression of sarcopenia in CKD. This counselling clinic should consist of an active clinical program situated in a medical fitness facility that specialized in dealing with chronic nephropathy. When patients first enter the program, they should be evaluated, after this evaluation, they should be counseled by a certified exercise physiologist who will prescribe an individualized exercise plan, which includes a combination of aerobic and resistance exercise. Then, nephrologists should make a revision of physical exercise for each individual to rule out possible contraindications for these patients. Finally, patients receive periodic motivational counseling, which includes review of the initial exercise prescription, identification of barriers to exercise, and reminder regarding patient's follow-up [8].

Anemia Treatment

A large multicenter cross-sectional study in stage 3–5 CKD performed by Finkelstein et al. showed that higher hemoglobin levels were associated with significantly higher HRQL scores, being the maximal score increase when hemoglobin ranges 10–12 g/dL, with blunted improvements above this level [13, 20].

Androgens

Testosterone deficiency is frequently present in male ESRD patients and is independently associated with adverse outcomes. In earlier stages of CKD, testosterone level was an independent predictor of muscle mass and strength, with low serum levels of testosterone in men which is a significant factor in the sarcopenia and frailty pathophysiology [12]. Since that testosterone has been proposed as a therapeutic alternative, if it is not contraindicated, to treating sarcopenic frailty older patients [10].

Vitamin D

Low 25-hydroxyvitamin D [25(OH)D] levels are associated with frailty in the older individuals. The vitamin acts directly on skeletal muscle influencing contractile muscle function and muscle metabolism. Gordon et al. demonstrated that 1,25(OH) D is a determinant of physical function and muscle size in CKD patients. Therefore, vitamin D deficiency may contribute to developing frailty in CKD, and this vitamin supplementation could be useful for treating this deficit [10, 12].

Other Measurements

Oral sodium bicarbonate treatment can be used to treat mild metabolic acidosis, improving nutritional parameters and muscle strength. Most guidelines currently recommend administering oral sodium bicarbonate when the serum bicarbonate concentration is <22 mmol/L, though the target of bicarbonatemia is not well-defined. It is also important to avoid periods of significant fluid overload that can stimulate the inflammatory cascade and subsequent protein catabolism, thus fluid restriction, diuretic therapy and RRT can be required. Finally, uremia leads to protein catabolism and subsequent sarcopenia, therefore the timing of dialysis initiation is important [12]. Angiotensin-converting enzyme inhibitors may improve the structure and biochemical function of skeletal muscle, and they may halt or slow senile decline in muscle strength. Other substances that may improve muscular function are growth hormone, androgens, and antioxidants [10]. In addition, avoidance of polypharmacy may be another efficient strategy to prevent or delay the onset of both frailty and sarcopenia [10, 12, 21].

There are a number of therapeutic options available for older CKD patients that should be chosen taking into consideration the patient's therapy choice and overall clinical functional status. These are nephroprevention strategies (conventional or modified), conservative treatment, dialysis initiation (early or delayed), or palliative care [4, 10, 22]. Regarding the conservative treatment, it has the objective of managing non-anuric ESRD patients without prescribing dialysis. It constitutes an alternative for handling non-terminal very old or frail older patients suffering from ESRD who are not adequate candidates for dialytic therapy, due to medical or personal (autonomy) reasons. For CKD conservative treatment many drugs can be used, such as loop diuretics for salt and water overload, potassium binders for hyperkalemia, subcutaneous erythropoietin for anemia, sodium bicarbonate for metabolic acidosis, activated charcoal for high serum urea, calcium supplements for hypocalcemia, and phosphate binders for hyperphosphatemia. Besides, this treatment also includes nutritionist counseling and psychological support [16].

Regarding the palliative treatment, which is used in terminal patients, consists of a symptomatic therapy (oxygen, analgesic, etc.) that includes psychological assistance [16]. In this regard, around 5% of older patients refuse to initiate dialysis and octogenarian patients may not be able to receive treatment due to extreme frailty, such as marked dementia or multiple comorbidities, due to lack of dialitic accesses or even intolerance to the procedure. On the contrary, withdrawal from dialysis is more frequent among nursing home dialysis patients, and discontinuation rate is associated to social and medical reasons, such as severe dementia or terminal oncological disease.

When senescent nephropathy is present, frailty treatment should be initiated based on its inducing condition. For example, whether muscle mass loss is identified as the patient's frailty-inducing factor, a normal diet and muscle exercise should be recommended, instead of a low-protein diet and low daily exercise. Moreover, the CKD therapeutic measures that are usually used should be executed more carefully in cases where frailty coexists with CKD, due to the patient's intolerance. In cases where conventional targets cannot be accomplished due to patient's intolerance to nephroprevention therapy, modified nephroprevention targets, doses ajusted to frailty, and more rigorous medical controls, should be sought (Table 11.4 and Fig. 11.1) [4].

References

1. Nixon AC, Bampouras TM, Pendleton N, Mitra S, Dhaygude AP. Diagnostic accuracy of frailty screening methods in advanced chronic kidney disease. Nephron. 2019;141(3):147–55. https://doi.org/10.1159/000494223.
2. Coppolino G, Bolignano D, Gareri P, Ruberto C, Andreucci M, Ruotolo G, Rocca M, Castagna A. Kidney function and cognitive decline in frail elderly: two faces of the same coin? Int Urol Nephrol. 2018;50(8):1505–10. https://doi.org/10.1007/s11255-018-1900-3.
3. Ali H, Abdelaal F, Baharani J. Assessment of frailty in elderly pre-dialysis population using simple tools. Saudi J Kidney Dis Transpl. 2017;28(4):716–24.
4. Ostuni M, Musso CG. Usefulness of frailty evaluation for handling chronic kidney disease elderly patients: a review and original proposal. Int Urol Nephrol. 2019;51(3):461–5. https://doi.org/10.1007/s11255-018-2061-0.
5. Demircioglu DT. The Association of Vitamin D levels and the frailty phenotype among non-geriatric dialysis patients: a cross-sectional study. Clinics (Sao Paulo). 2018;73:e116. https://doi.org/10.6061/clinics/2018/e116.

6. Musso CG, Vilas M, Onuigbo M. Nephroprevention in the oldest old with chronic kidney disease: special considerations. World J Nephrol. 2015;4(1):1–5. https://doi.org/10.5527/wjn.v4.i1.1.
7. Adame Perez SI, Senior PA, Field CJ, Jindal K, Mager DR. Frailty, health-related quality of life, cognition, depression, vitamin D and health-care utilization in an ambulatory adult population with type 1 or type 2 diabetes mellitus and chronic kidney disease: a cross-sectional analysis. Can J Diabetes. 2019;43(2):90–7. https://doi.org/10.1016/j.jcjd.2018.06.001.
8. Bohm CJ, Storsley LJ, Hiebert BM, Nelko S, Tangri N, Cheskin LJ, McAdams-DeMarco MA, Rigatto C. Impact of exercise counseling on physical function in chronic kidney disease: an observational study. Can J Kidney Health Dis. 2018;5:2054358117753615. https://doi.org/10.1177/2054358117753615.
9. Van Pilsum Rasmussen S, Konel J, Warsame F, Ying H, Buta B, Haugen C, King E, DiBrito S, Varadhan R, Rodríguez-Mañas L, Walston JD, Segev DL, McAdams-DeMarco M. Engaging clinicians and patients to assess and improve frailty measurement in adults with end stage renal disease. BMC Nephrol. 2018;19(1):8. https://doi.org/10.1186/s12882-017-0806-0.
10. Musso CG, Jauregui JR, Macías Núñez JF. Frailty phenotype and chronic kidney disease: a review of the literature. Int Urol Nephrol. 2015;47(11):1801–7. https://doi.org/10.1007/s11255-015-1112-z.
11. McAdams-DeMarco MA, Ying H, Thomas AG, Warsame F, Shaffer AA, Haugen C, Garonzik-Wang JM, Desai NM, Varadhan R, Walston J, Norman SP, Segev DL. Frailty, inflammatory markers, and waitlist mortality among patients with end-stage renal disease in a prospective cohort study. Transplantation. 2018;102(10):1740–6. https://doi.org/10.1097/TP.0000000000002213.
12. Nixon AC, Bampouras TM, Pendleton N, Woywodt A, Mitra S, Dhaygude A. Frailty and chronic kidney disease: current evidence and continuing uncertainties. Clin Kidney J. 2018;11(2):236–45. https://doi.org/10.1093/ckj/sfx134.
13. Kittiskulnam P, Sheshadri A, Johansen K. Consequences of CKD on functioning. Semin Nephrol. 2016;36(4):305–18. https://doi.org/10.1016/j.semnephrol.2016.05.007.
14. Kamijo, Kanda E, Ishibashi Y, Yoshida M. Sarcopenia and frailty in PD: impact on mortality, malnutrition, and inflammation. Perit Dial Int. 2018;38(6):447–54. https://doi.org/10.3747/pdi.2017.00271.
15. McAdams-DeMarco MA, Ying H, Olorundare I, King EA, Desai N, Dagher N, Lonze B, Montgomery R, Walston J, Segev DL. Frailty and health-related quality of life in end stage renal disease patients of all ages. J Frailty Aging. 2016;5(3):174–9.
16. Musso CG, Trigka K, Dousdampanis P, Jauregui J. Therapeutic alternatives and palliative care for advanced renal disease in the very elderly: a review of the literature. Int Urol Nephrol. 2015;47(4):647–54. https://doi.org/10.1007/s11255-014-0886-8.
17. Ortiz A, Sanchez-niño M. Sarcopenia in CKD: a roadmap from basic pathogenetic mechanisms to clinical trials. Clin Kidney J. 2019;12(1):110–2.
18. Sieverdes JC, Rao V, Taber DJ, Noltemeyer Z, McGillicuddy JW, Bergamin M, Thangavel S, Baliga PK. Feasibility and functional testing for frailty in chronic kidney disease. Prog Transplant. 2018;28(3):299–300. https://doi.org/10.1177/1526924818781577.
19. Moffatt H, Moorhouse P, Mallery L, Landry D, Tennankore K. Using the Frailty Assessment for Care Planning Tool (FACT) to screen elderly chronic kidney disease patients for frailty: the nurse experience. Clin Interv Aging. 2018;13:843–52. https://doi.org/10.2147/CIA.S150673.
20. Wawer AA, Jennings A, Fairweather-Tait SJ. Iron status in the elderly: a review of recent evidence. Mech Ageing Dev. 2018;175:55–73. https://doi.org/10.1016/j.mad.2018.07.003.
21. Formica M, Politano P, Marazzi F, Tamagnone M, Serra I, Marengo M, Falconi D, Gherzi M, Tattoli F, Bottaro C, Giuliano D, Tibaldi V, Isaia GC. Acute kidney injury and chronic kidney disease in the elderly and polypharmacy. Blood Purif. 2018;46(4):332–6. https://doi.org/10.1159/000492149.
22. Bansal AD, Leonberg-Yoo A, Schell JO, Scherer JS, Jones CA. Ten tips nephrologists wish the palliative care team knew about caring for patients with kidney disease. J Palliat Med. 2018;21(4):546–51. https://doi.org/10.1089/jpm.2018.0087.

Chapter 12
Frailty in Older Dialysis Patients

Adina Carmen Ilie, Andra Nastasa, Victoria Paula Musso-Enz, Carlos Guido Musso, and Adrian Covic

Aging, CKD, and Frailty

In the future, the share of older individuals ($\geq$ 65 years) is projected to increase; for example, it is anticipated that the percent of this category in the total population of the European Union will rise from 19.2% at the start of 2016 to 29.1% by 2080 [1]. On the other hand, chronic kidney disease (CKD) is a growing problem among older people, with an increasing prevalence due to socio-economic development and better life expectancy.

The older dialysis population is also expanding, as shown by numerous data: in Dialysis Outcomes and Practice Patterns (DOPPS) study, the mean age of participants at study entry increased over time in all 12 DOPPS countries. Also, older patients

A. C. Ilie
University of Medicine and Pharmacy Grigore T. Popa, Iasi, Romania

Division of Geriatric Medicine & Gerontology, Dr.C.I. Parhon Hospital, Iasi, Romania

A. Nastasa · A. Covic
University of Medicine and Pharmacy Grigore T. Popa, Iasi, Romania

Nephrology Division, Dr.C.I. Parhon Hospital, Iasi, Romania

V. P. Musso-Enz
Physiology Department, Instituto Universitario del Hospital Italiano de Buenos Aires, Buenos Aires, Argentina

C. G. Musso (✉)
Physiology Department, Instituto Universitario del Hospital Italiano de Buenos Aires, Buenos Aires, Argentina

Nephrology Division, Hospital Italiano de Buenos Aires, Buenos Aires, Argentina

Facultad de Ciencias de la Salud, Universidad Simón Bolívar, Barranquilla, Colombia

Ageing Biology Unit, Hospital Italiano de Buenos Aires, Buenos Aires, Argentina
e-mail: carlos.musso@hospitalitaliano.org.ar

© Springer Nature Switzerland AG 2021

C. G. Musso et al. (eds.), *Frailty and Kidney Disease*,
https://doi.org/10.1007/978-3-030-53529-2_12

represented a different proportion of DOPPS participants across countries and regions with the highest percentage of very old dialysis patients (≥75 years) in Europe (27.4%) [2]. The increase of the older patients in dialysis based on the expansion of the population 70 years of age and older is a trend also observed in Japan [3] and the USA [4].

With the growing number of older patients with recognized CKD, the issue of frailty appears to be of major interest because both aging and CKD share this common feature. Moreover, CKD accelerates the process of aging via protein energy wasting, uremic toxins, and chronic inflammation [5]. The combined consequences of chronological and pathological aging may explain the higher prevalence of frailty in CKD patients.

Normal aging should be distinguished from pathological aging (senescence) since the latter characteristically reduces the homeostatic capability of older people, making them frail. Additionally, CKD is associated to deleterious processes (inflammation, oxidative stress, protein-energy wasting, etc.) which accelerate and worsen the aging process inducing fragility [6, 7]. Moreover, coexistence of frailty and CKD has been documented to increase risks of falls, fractures, hospitalization, and mortality [8]. Therefore, there is a deteriorating interdependence between CKD and aging where CKD makes aging accelerate and worsen (senescence), while senescence makes CKD accelerate its deterioration (senescent nephropathy), with frailty status being the common path which catalyzes this spiral of damage. Frail older CKD patients suffer from a condition that has been called *senescent nephropathy*, which usually has different clinical complications, therapeutic needs, and worse overall prognosis compared to fit CKD older patients (chronic nephropathy). Consequently, older dialysis patients should be evaluated in order to identify the presence of frailty, and when frailty status is documented, rehabilitation therapy should be added to their dialytic treatment. In addition, conventional dialysis targets, if not tolerated, should be adapted to the patient's frailty status [9].

An important aspect that needs to be underlined is that prevalence estimates are affected by the way frailty is assessed. Although definition or the diagnostic criteria of "frailty" have not gained broad consensus, there are two main approaches to assess physical frailty: the first, Cumulative Deficit Model, consists of summing together an individual's number of conditions and impairments to create a Frailty Index [10]. The second model was originally defined by Fried et al. [11] as a Phenotype Model of Frailty consisting of at least three of the following five components: unintentional weight loss, exhaustion, physical inactivity, slow gait speed, and weak grip strength. In order to apply the notion of frailty to patients with CKD or end-stage renal disease (ESRD), the frailty phenotype has been adapted in numerous ways, but still remained anchored to the five domains initially established by Fried et al. Using the customized criteria for application to NHANES III data, Wilhelm-Leen et al. [12] found that frailty was significantly associated with all stages of CKD and particularly with moderate to severe CKD, even after adjustment for the residual effects of age, sex, race, and prevalent chronic diseases; in other words, risk of frailty was increased approximately two-fold in mild CKD and approximately six-fold in persons with moderate to severe CKD (at an estimated glomerular filtration rate <45 mL/min/1.73 m^2, prevalence of frailty was 20.9%).

Frailty is more prevalent among patients on hemodialysis (HD), varying between 14% and 73% [13], as a result of heterogeneity between the methods used to assess it. When using a self-report-based definition of frailty in a cohort of 2275 dialyzed adults, Johansen et al. found that two-thirds of the patients were frail and that older age, female sex, and HD (rather than peritoneal dialysis) were independently associated with frailty [14]. The substantially higher prevalence of frailty among ESRD patients could be explained by the fact that worsening kidney function is associated with many of the same clinical features as advanced age in the absence of kidney disease, such as loss of muscle mass, inactivity, high burden of comorbid conditions, and decline in physical and cognitive functioning.

The fact that frailty is extremely common among dialysis patients raises the next question about its significance. There is strong evidence that links frailty with an increased risk of death, hospitalization, falls, and fractures [13]; in an attempt to quantify the association of frailty with adverse outcomes of mortality and hospitalization in 146 prevalent HD patients, McAdams-deMarco et al. found that the 3-year mortality was 40% for frail participants, compared with 16% for non-frail [15]. The proportion with two or more hospitalizations over the subsequent year after enrollment was 43% for frail patients, compared with 28% for non-frail hemodialysis-dependent adults [15]. An additional study [16] found that frailty independently predicted a threefold higher number of falls in a cohort of 95 hemodialysis patients, regardless of age.

Frailty impacts not only clinical outcomes, but also the patient-centered outcome of health-related quality of life (HRQOL). In a prospective study of 233 patients with ESRD, participants who were frail at the initial assessment were 2.91-fold more likely to report worse HRQOL at follow-up [17]; this observation highlights frail ESRD patients as a highly vulnerable population that is significantly impacted by their health status.

Given the relationship between frailty and adverse outcomes, greater attention should be focused on identifying frail dialysis patients and on creating an adequate strategy to address frailty, including managing risk factors that may exacerbate its progression.

Even though it has been reported that two-thirds of the incident dialysis patients are frail, and within the first 6 months, more than 30% of them usually have functional loss requiring caregiver support or transfer to a nursing home, almost two-thirds of older patients can perform peritoneal dialysis (PD) on their own. This phenomenon has been attributed to the fact that cognitive tests usually show better performance for older patients on PD than on HD [18, 19].

Risk Factors for Frailty in Older HD Patients

Accelerated Aging

Frailty is a geriatric syndrome, being first described in the older population. In the hemodialysis (HD) population, frailty is also described in non-older HD population. Since aging is described as an important factor associated with frailty [20], in HD population accelerated aging is involved [21]. Dialysis patients might age

15 years faster as described in the Gomperts equation model. [22] Factors involved in accelerated aging are multiple and divers: chronic inflammation, oxidative stress, angiotensin II (AT-II), cardiovascular disease and risk factors, S-Klotho, the sirtuins (SIRT), and the target of rapamycin (TOR).

Uremia and CKD are characterized by activation of immunity, which is characterized by activated monocytes and increased synthesis of proinflammatory cytokines (IL- 6, tumor necrosis factor [TNF], and IL- 1) and chemokines [20]. Also, in advanced CKD, there is an impaired removal of proinflammatory cytokines and exposure to inflammatory stimulants such as uremic toxins and even toxins produced by the dialysis procedure itself. Moreover, aging itself predisposes to chronic inflammation [22, 23]. Inflammation in HD patients is contributing to frailty through multiple ways: anorexia, malnutrition and protein-energy wasting, muscle wasting, protein degradation, insulin resistance, among others [24, 25].

Oxidative stress and free radicals are increasing both with age and with CKD, and are involved in inflammation, accelerated aging and frailty in HD patients [26, 27]. Advanced glycation end products are the result of oxidative stress and have been implicated in healthy, age-related reduction in kidney function and are certainly accelerated in HD patients [27].

AT-II receptors (ATR) are involved in normal aging. ATR-1 stimulation promotes mitochondrial damage and reactive oxygen species production leading to age related vascular changes. Opposite, ATR-2 promotes vasodilatation [28]. In HD patients, ATR-1 expression is significantly increased, compared to non-dialyzed patients, leading to increasing of the intrarenal renin-angiotensin system (RAS) activation and to subsequent renal damage. Modifications occur even after initiation of dialysis [29].

Cardiovascular disease and risk factors are involved in accelerated age-related decline in renal function in older patients [28]. HD frail, older patients, are more likely to have diabetes mellitus and cardiovascular conditions, including congestive heart failure, coronary artery disease or myocardial infarction, cerebrovascular accident or transient ischemia attack, peripheral vascular disease, and other cardiac disease [30]. Also, classical predictors of frailty such as decreased muscular strength and muscle mass and the cardiovascular disease were observed in older HD patients with frailty [21]. Peripheral artery disease is closely associated with frailty in HD patients and low grip strength, and the small thigh circumference values are significantly associated with the existence of peripheral artery disease [31].

The relationship between Klotho, one of the most powerful aging-suppressor gene, and renal function is an inverse one, and has been previously documented. Klotho deficiency might exacerbate hyperphosphatemia in uremic patients, leading to further accelerated inflammation and increasing vascular calcification [32]. Moreover, in HD older male patients, low plasma S-klotho levels are related to impaired physical performance [33], marker for sarcopenia and frailty.

SIRT-1 is another longevity gene involved both in renal aging and frailty. SIRT-1 under-expression promotes pro-fibrotic and pro-apoptotic effects in renal interstitial cells leading to accelerated aging [28]. Moreover, in hemodialyzed patients, SIRT-1 polymorphisms are associated with abnormal cholesterol metabolism and coronary artery calcification [34], factors for frailty in older HD patients.

In community-dwelling older adults, frailty is associated with elevated markers of systemic inflammation, particularly interleukin-6, soluble tumor necrosis factor-receptor-1 and C-reactive protein. This is illustrated by a multi-center study of 762 hemodialysis patients, in whom increased interleukin-6 levels were associated with an increase in the Fried frailty phenotype score [35].

Sarcopenia

Sarcopenia in older HD patients is an important determinant for frailty. Older patients on HD are exposed to conditions related to the disease (increased protein catabolism induced by metabolic acidosis, pro-inflammatory cytokines, hyperparathyroidism, associated diseases), related to the dialysis procedure (increased protein degradation and reduced protein synthesis, dialysis nutrient loss) and related to subsequent protein energy wasting and mechanical changes, all of which predispose them to an important loss of muscle mass and muscle strength [36]. Besides, sarcopenia is usually related to malnutrition-inflammation-atherosclerosis (MIA) syndrome in dialysis patients [37], and it can be quantified through muscle mass and muscle strength [38, 39]. Most commonly used measures for sarcopenia are dual energy x-ray absorptiometry, bioelectrical impedance, sum of skinfold thicknesses, calf circumference and mid-arm muscle circumference and muscle strength evaluated by handgrip dynamometer and decreased physical function evaluated by walking speed [36]. Lamarca et al. conducted a study to identify sarcopenia in older HD patients using different measures. They found that the prevalence of sarcopenia varied from 3.9% to 63.3% and only 2–15.7% of the patients were classified as sarcopenic by more than two diagnostic criteria, suggesting a low rate of agreement among these [36]. Different data reported a 31.5% prevalence of sarcopenia in older HD patients and the diagnosis of sarcopenia was mainly driven by muscle mass measurement because muscle strength was low in the large majority of HD patients [40]. Sarcopenic obesity and its presence in older HD patients is known to increase chronic inflammation and the risk of falls [41, 42]. Bao et al. found in the Comprehensive Dialysis Study that higher estimated GFR at dialysis initiation was associated with higher odds of frailty. Since GFR estimation was based on creatininemia, a high estimated GFR value may reflect in fact sarcopenia. In addition, the uremic symptoms that led nephrologists to prescribe dialysis initiation to these patients could be in fact symptoms of frailty phenotype [43]. Sarcopenia is characteristically associated with all-cause mortality, and it is usually documented in 10.9% of PD patients, a proportion that is lower than the one reported in HD patients. Even though nutritional assessment is very important in all dialysis patients, it is particularly crucial in frail older patients who have high peritoneal protein loss in order to avoid worsening sarcopenia [37, 44].

Malnutrition

Incidence of malnutrition varies in the older HD patients, depending on the measurement tool used. One study documented that 4% of the patients were malnourished and almost half (47%) of the patients were at risk for malnutrition [45]. Another set of data also shows a highly variable prevalence of malnutrition or protein-energy wasting (PEW), ranging from 26% to 77% in the older dialysis population depending on the methods used to define it [46]. The methods used for determining malnutrition or PEW in older HD patients vary from screening tests such as Mini Nutritional Assessment (MNA), malnutrition inflammation score (MIS), subjective global assessment (SGA), to biochemical data such as albumin and pre-albumin levels, to corporal composition. Causes for malnutrition in older HD patients are: age-related (reduced metabolic expenditure, anorexia, low muscle mass and function, sedentarism, taste abnormalities), psychosocial and medical-related factors (dementia, depression, comorbidity, polypharmacy, poverty, loneliness, dependency), and CKD factors (uremic toxicity, metabolic derangements, inflammation-related catabolism, dialysis-related catabolism, dysregulation of gastrointestinal homeostatic mechanisms, altered blood concentration of appetite regulators, and deranged hypothalamic output) [47, 48]. Older HD patients also have poor dietary quality and higher consumption of processed and ultra-processed food, and these dietary negative habits are exacerbated during dialysis days. The factors involved are multiple dietary restrictions which might lead to a poorer overall dietary quality, consisting of a lower intake of fiber, vitamins, and nutrients that ultimately falls outside of what is generally recommended as a healthy diet [49]. In older HD patients, we must rethink the benefits of dietary restrictions regarding the overall health of dialyzed patients and regarding the higher risk for malnutrition, and subsequent frailty with their important adverse outcomes. Regarding obesity, it improves survival in dialysis patients (reverse epidemiology), a phenomenon that can be explained by the fact that progressive wasting and chronic inflammation outweigh the influence of traditional cardiovascular risk factors. Therefore, evaluating parameters of body composition, such as mid-arm muscle circumference (lean mass surrogate) and triceps-skinfold thickness (fat mass surrogate), can also be useful in evaluating all-cause mortality risk in dialysis patients [43]. Regarding nutritional status in PD older patients, they have better scores in the subjective global nutritional assessment, compared to those patients on HD. This may be due to the significant caloric contribution that this modality provides to patients (300–450 kilocalories / day). This constitutes a nutritional advantage, as long as it does not lead to being overweight or is not associated with a significant protein loss. Thus, it is essential that the patient has adequate nutritional control, particularly in this population [19, 50–52].

Depression

Frailty has not only a physical compound, but also a social and mental compound, and depression is an important factor in frailty. Frailty and depression share several risk factors, such as chronic inflammation, oxidative stress, mitochondrial dysfunction, hypothalamic-pituitary axis dysregulation, and vascular disease, all with higher frequency in older HD patients [53].

Recent data shows that 31% of the older HD patients had symptoms of depression [52] leading to increased frailty and to negative outcomes. The extended Frail and Elderly Patients on Dialysis (FEPOD) emphasizes the fact that older patient on HD have lower depression score compared with patients with conservative kidney management. Moreover, in this study, worsening frailty was associated with higher depression scores underlining the strong connection between depression and frailty [54].

Cognitive Decline

There is a causal link between frailty and cognitive impairment in older HD patients, and age-associated processes that lead to frailty are also responsible for cognitive decline. The mechanisms involved in cognitive impairment and subsequent frailty comprises inflammation, cardiovascular disease, nutrition, neuropathology, and the effect of uremic toxins [55]. Prevalence of cognitive impairment in older HD patients ranges from 6% to 13%, depending on the measurement test and may reach 41% in the very old persons [56]. Cognitive impairment and frailty are significantly associated with a higher risk of adverse health outcomes such as mortality, dependence, institutionalization, among others [57]. New data about frailty and cognitive decline in HD older patients will be available after the completion of The Cognitive decline in Older Patients with End stage renal disease (COPE) study, which has multiple objectives, including to determine the underlying pathophysiological mechanisms [58]. Wolfgram et al. documented that those patients who began their dialysis therapy with the peritoneal modality had a 25% lower risk of acquiring dementia compared to those who did it with HD, despite adjusting for risk factors such as age and diabetes mellitus. It has been postulated that fluctuations in blood volume and blood pressure that occur during HD could lead to repeated episodes of cerebral ischemia [59].

Cardiovascular Complications

Hemodialysis can have significantly negative circulatory impact on older patients, particularly in frail ones [60]. This hemodynamic effect is especially notable at the level of coronary flow, causing a transient abnormality in the movement of the heart wall known as "myocardial stunning," which after repeated hemodialytic sessions can lead to fixed defects, and finally, systolic cardiac dysfunction and heart failure. This cardiac abnormality during the hemodialysis session has a strong correlation with age and at the same time is associated with premature death [61, 62]. Moreover, preexisting cardiac dysfunction in the frail older population can cause arrhythmias, hypotension, and the sensation of marked post-dialysis asthenia [19, 63]. Conversely, peritoneal dialysis has an advantage over HD, since it does not cause such hemodynamic insult and therefore does not induce "myocardial stunning," which makes it a more reasonable option for older adult patients with lower coronary reserve [61, 62]. Therefore, it has been reported that survival would be slightly higher in frail patients who started PD compared to those patients who started HD, phenomenon which could be explained because of lower risk of cardiovascular complications in the peritoneal modality [60].

Consequences of Frailty in Older Dialysis Patients

Falls

Falls are common in the older HD patients and represent a marker of underlying frailty and functional dependence. The FEPOD study showed that of 47% of older dialyzed patients experienced at least one fall during 2-year follow-up, and this data was comparable between PD and HD. Moreover, having one or more previous falls was associated with a 2.5 times higher risk of new falls [64]. The predisposing factors for falls in older HD patients are multiple and frailty with its sarcopenia is a major one. More cited factors are: mineral and bone disorder associated to CKD [65], presence of multiple comorbidities at the time of starting dialysis, including a high prevalence of diabetes mellitus, cardiovascular disease, depression, sleep disorders, restless leg syndrome, and peripheral and autonomic neuropathies, multiple medication [66]. There are also factors related to HD such as marked fluid, electrolyte and weight shifts during dialysis therapy may represent unique risk factors in dialysis patients who are prone to dizziness, hypotension, and arrhythmias in the post-dialysis period [67]. After one episode of fall, the fear caused by falling is leading to limitation of activities and leaving the home less frequently. This inactivity due to fear of falling may lead to decreased strength, agility, and balance, which will lead to further loss of independence, further functional decline, and subsequent falling [43].

Peritoneal dialysis allows dialysis treatment to be carried out in the comfort of the home, as well as avoiding transfer to the dialysis unit several times a week, thus it is a less stressful dialytic modality for dialysis patients suffering from gait disorder and increased risk of falls. This fact contributes to give these patient the opportunity of not having to depend on a family member or an ambulance to move [61, 62]. Additionally, by avoiding transportation, frail patients can invest this time in their physical rehabilitation [61, 68]. Lower mobility associated to frailty phenotype, can represent an advantage in older peritoneal dialysis patients since this reduced physical activity leads to less frequent exit-site complications [45]. Information technologies such as telenephrology, recording and monitoring devices, make handling frail older PD patients at home much simpler, reducing their need of visiting dialysis units [69].

Hospitalizations

The number of hospitalization episodes has been considered a sign of poor clinical prognosis, which are associated with frailty. The rate of visits to hospital emergency services among frail older HD patients is almost twice that of non-frail patients and the mean hospital stay is longer [70]. Similar data are described in other studies, where hospitalizations were associated with frailty and falls, and hospitalization rate was 2–2.5 times higher compared to non-frail older HD patients [55, 71].

Dependence/Disability

In older HD patients, severely impaired performance status ranged from 13% to 33%, depended by modality of diagnosis and population [53]. In the study conducted by Kurella Tamura et al. investigating functional status of older adults before and after initiation of dialysis, the results showed that within 3 months after the start of dialysis, 61% of the older patients had died or had a decrease in functional status as compared with their functional status before dialysis, and 39% had the same functional status that they had before dialysis. Moreover, by 12 months, 87% of older HD patients had died or had a decrease in functional status [72]. Impaired mobility appears to be the strong indicator for early mortality among all clinical risk factors, including calendar age and comorbidity, with total dependency for transfers being independently associated with 3-month mortality, as described in REIN registry [73]. All expressions of disability such as dependence for transfers, dependence in Activities of Daily Living, and impaired mobility were associated with mortality in older, frail, HD patients [53].

Decreased Quality of Life (QoL)

QoL in patients on dialysis treatment is worse than that of a general population comparable for age and gender, despite the dialysis type. Associated frailty has a significant negative role on physical component of QoL that is more compromised than the mental one and dependence is also having a significant negative effect on many domains of QoL [74]. Newer data confirmed that dialysis modality was not significantly associated with measures of QoL, but higher frailty scores were associated with lower QoL, even after adjustment for dialysis modality and other patient characteristics [75]. Data from the FEPOD study showed that treatment by dialysis, both with peritoneal dialysis and HD, improved some QoL measures, but overall, PD was slightly better than the other modalities in the older population. However, as in the primary FEPOD study, frailty was associated with worse

QoL measures [48]. Studies in the United Kingdom showed no differences in QoL, survival, or the need for hospitalizations between patients on PD and HD. This was also observed with respect to the SF-12 score, although the mental domain score favored patients on PD, especially after the first year of renal replacement therapy [62, 76]. This is probably linked to the fact that the method rating as intrusive is significantly higher for HD than for PD [62, 63, 68]. Although some studies reported no significant differences in the QoL among older patients on HD and non-assisted PD, other studies did document a better QoL in older patients treated with assisted PD versus HD. Perhaps, this difference could be explained by a different fragility status among the studied patients [19, 63, 77].

Increasing Healthcare Costs

In older, frail HD patients with multiple comorbidities and multiple consequences of frailty, the hospitalizations are multiple, with higher lengths and also the visits to the emergency department are frequent. The number of visits to the emergency service and hospitalizations are important information for the management of healthcare resources. This may lead to saturation of these services and increasing healthcare costs [46]. Also, the healthcare costs are increasing due to the increasing need for assistance associated with altered functional status of older HD patients and due to increasing need for institutionalization, medical chronical services, other than dialysis and multiple medications. It is worth pointing out that PD allows dialysis treatment to be carried out at home, as well as avoiding transfer to the dialysis unit several times a week, helping consequently to save resources [61, 63].

Death

The older frail HD patients have a high burden of comorbid illness, leading to a high overall mortality. However, frailty has been found to be independently associated with higher mortality in all studies that have examined the association between frailty and mortality [78]. Newer data about mortality in older HD patients are described by van Loon et al. and showed that the 2-year mortality rate is 29% [55]. Mortality rates in older, frail patients are influenced by multiple factors: fall, depression, impaired mobility, age, cognitive status, clinical status before dialysis initiation, social factors, presences of family, institutionalization, and more to be investigated.

How to Approach an Older, Frail HD Patient

Comprehensive Geriatric Assessment (CGA)

The management of frailty involves an integrated approach. From this point of view, CGA emerges as an important step, because it represents a model of care based on a multidisciplinary assessment that identifies medical, psychosocial, functional, and environmental needs, and informs development of a coordinated care plan [79].

CGA is widely used in geriatric care, but not often applied outside this spectrum; most evidence for its effectiveness derives from acute hospital settings, where a systematic assessment has been associated with better outcomes in terms of physical function and survival [80]. Although the role of CGA in chronic disease settings is less well established, growing data suggest that it is feasible to use it within nephrology care, with the mention of further research required in order to assess outcomes [81, 82].

Components of CGA that are most relevant to managing geriatric patients with ESRD on dialysis are: functional status assessment (estimated by determining a patient's ability to perform routine tasks of daily life or Activities of Daily Living – ADL), cognitive impairment assessment (using tools like "MoCA" test for evaluation of executive dysfunction), nutritional analysis, and also identification of other important issues like polypharmacy, depression, risk of falls [83]. It has been suggested that the CGA should take place at the moment of dialysis initiation and at any major change in a patient's health or functional status (such as hospitalization), in order to re-evaluate the management plan [83].

Identifying dialyzed patients at risk of functional disability and/or decline with the help of CGA may have the potential to maximize health outcome priorities for patients: rehabilitation and maintenance of independence [84].

Nutrition

Nutrition is a greater challenge in the older than in the younger dialysis patients because there are several factors that can interfere with maintaining adequate nutritional status, like decreased mobility, impaired cognitive function, reduced appetite. Taken together, these factors contribute to the concept of undernutrition, which has a major impact on the development of sarcopenia and frailty [85]. A recent study conducted by Villain et al. on 3165 incident HD patients ≥75 years of age from 178 French dialysis units showed that poor nutritional status was the variable most strongly associated with mortality, with a negative prognostic impact of low nutritional markers [86]. This finding represents a consolidation of the statement outlined by the guidelines that "preserving nutritional status should prevail over any other dietary restriction" [87].

In order to maintain an adequate nutritional status in the frail older dialysis patient, the first matter that needs to be addressed is identification of possible causes for reduced appetite; these can include medication, metabolic acidosis, intercurrent illness, and comorbid conditions such as depression [88]. Secondary, the dietary advice should consider that the risks of undernutrition and protein energy wasting may outweigh the benefits of rigorous phosphate control in the frail cohort, demanding more individualized and "relaxed" dietary restrictions in this context [87].

Regarding nutritional requirements for older patients, there are some directions stated by the guidelines: according to Kidney Disease Outcomes Quality Initiative (KDOQI) guideline, the recommended energy intake for patients ≥60 years of age undergoing maintenance HD is 30 kcal/kg/day [30]. The protein requirements are not differentiated with regard to age by the renal nutritional guidelines for dialysis, which recommend a higher protein intake for all adults, ranging from 1.1 to 1.4 g/kg/day [89–93].

Individualized Physical Activity

Maintenance HD patients display reduced levels of daily physical activity, and this is associated with poorer physical performance [94] and lower survival rates [95]. Since physical inactivity is part of the definition of frailty, interventions that increase activity have the potential to attenuate frailty. Recognized as a feasible measure of treatment, exercise intervention counteracts muscle-wasting in CKD patients and can be implemented safely in the ESRD population [96, 97]. Numerous studies have shown that regular exercise has a positive impact on physical and mental component, QoL, and survival [98, 99]. Both aerobic and resistance exercise interventions, administered in the dialysis facility (intradialytic) or outside of dialysis (interdialytic), have the potential to improve physical performance, cognitive function and even contribute to a better quality of social interaction [100].

The concept of geriatric rehabilitation in the dialysis population involves a therapeutic intervention whose purpose is to restore functional ability or enhance residual functional capability in those with disabling impairments [101]. Within a rehabilitative framework, physical rehabilitation plays a major role, but psychosocial intervention, cognitive rehabilitation, and environmental modification are also important [102]. For frail older adults on dialysis, the exercise demands must be lowered and such an intervention may seem more difficult to implement. If there is appropriate consideration of the individual patient's medical condition and functional needs, it is conceivable that increasing physical activity in this special population may improve frailty. In rehabilitation models for geriatric dialysis population, the concept of interdisciplinarity is mandatory, requiring a team including doctors, nurses, physiotherapists, psychologists, and dieticians [102]. A large study of inpatient rehabilitation for HD patients [103] included 164 individuals with a mean age of 74.5 years, with functional limitations (new-onset disability from prolonged illness or an acute event rendering them incapable of living independently). The management strategy included physical and/or cognitive exercises performed twice a day and lasting from 30 to 60 minutes per session, short daily dialysis sessions (2 hours 6 times weekly) in order to limit interference with rehabilitation sessions and liberalized renal diets to improve nutritional balance and participation; after a median of 48.5 days, a substantial proportion of patients (69%) achieved meaningful improvement in functional independence scores and could be discharged to their homes, proving the feasibility of an integrated dialysis rehabilitation service [103].

Other rehabilitation models include home-based programs (with risk of lower adherence rates) or targeted interventions to reduce the risk of falls (by amplifying patient's awareness, staff education, implementation of fall risk assessment tools, and simple environmental modifications) [104]. A 14-week intradialytic training program can induce significant improvements on physical performance. However, the rate of clinically meaningful responders is low and the level of responsiveness depends on baseline physical status, highlighting the need to individualize exercise prescription [105].

How to Approach an Older, Frail PD Patient

Assisted PD

Since there is more frailty status and comorbidities in older dialysis patients, they usually suffer from cognitive impairment, vision impairment, deafness, and/or limited mobility, which are all conditions that affect the ideal operating framework for applying PD. Hence, frail PD patients usually need the assisted modality [61, 63, 68, 77]. In addition, data from registries show that older patients who choose assisted PD have longer survival time compared to those patients who perform self-dialysis [45], and even the risk of peritonitis seems to be lower in older individuals dialyzed by assisted modality compared to young adults on self-peritoneal dialysis [106, 107]. However, it should be taken into account that even though training frail older individuals in the PD technique can take more time compared to the young adult, this does not mean that they cannot perform their own peritoneal dialysis [61, 68].

Residual Diuresis

Non-conventional dialytic modalities (incremental, functional, or palliative dialysis), which are explained in detail at the end of this chapter, are usually less stressful in frail older dialysis patients since they imply shorter time or lower speed pump HD sessions, or lower dialysis volumes and/or exchange number in PD. However, these modalities can be better applied if patient's residual diuresis is preserved. In this sense, PD allows greater conservation of residual renal function compared to

HD. This advantage has been attributed to the significantly lower ischemic kidney damage induced by the PD [61, 76].

Dialytic Adequacy in Frail Older Patients

Early dialysis initiation (GFR: 10 ml/min/1.73 m^2) in very old patients was found to be associated with greater rate of mortality and hospitalization. However, other studies documented that survival was reduced in patients starting dialysis at GFR: 6 ml/min/1.73 m^2, compared with those patients starting dialysis earlier. Perhaps, these different findings could reflect differences in their frailty status among the studied groups. Even though how dialysis initiation affects frailty is not fully understood yet, it appears that neither frailty status nor disability improved after starting dialysis [18].

Although dialysis seems to prolong longevity in older individuals compared to conservative treatment, it does not in the sickest older patients. Some authors have reported a loss of independence in very old end-stage renal disease patients who started dialysis, observing that many patients deteriorate their functional state at 3 months from the beginning of the treatment, becoming frailer and sarcopenic, since they have fewer activities which are limited by the time spent on dialysis and their post-dialysis fatigue. In these cases, conservative treatment could be a better therapeutic alternative. In addition, an association between frailty status and increased GFR at starting dialysis is documented, phenomenon which could be explained on one hand, because signs and symptoms of frailty could be assumed as secondary to uremia, leading to an earlier onset of dialysis. On the other hand, GFR could be overestimated in these patients since their creatininemia is relatively lower because of their sarcopenia. Thus, in order to determine the best time to initiate dialysis, it would be important to consider factors other than the nephrological ones (GFR, electrolyte levels, etc.), and frailty status should also be included in this assessment. When dialysis seems to be a beneficial therapeutic alternative in this population, a GFR between 7 and 9 ml/min/1.73 m^2 could be an adequate time for starting dialysis in clinical and laboratory stable end-stage renal disease oldest old patients [108]. Regarding which would be the best dialytic modality for older people, many reports showed a reasonable survival on HD or PD. However, it is worth mentioning that most of octogenarians end-stage renal disease patients opt for renal replacement treatment when dialysis is deemed appropriate by their nephrologists. Consequently, these older patients usually rely their treatment decisions more on their health care team, having the risk that the modality favored by their nephrologists will become their treatment of choice [8]. Since frail individuals are highly prevalent among this aged group, and around 60% of them require some sort of assistance, home assisted dialysis (PD or HD) appears to be an adequate dialytic option for them. Very old patients who are not able for self-care can be supported through assisted dialysis, mainly assisted PD, where trained caregivers provide daily dialysis assistance either in a nursing home or at the patient's home [61, 68]. Kurella Tamura et al. examined the effect of dialysis initiation on functional status, measured by the degree of dependence in activities of daily living; 12 months after starting chronic dialysis, 58% of these patients had died and their predialysis functional status had been maintained in only 13% of them, thus finding that dialysis initiation was associated with an abrupt decline in patients´ functional status [18]. In addition, other authors also documented a loss of independent function 1 year after initiation of long-term dialysis in oldest old end-stage renal disease patients who suffered from multiple conditions. At dialysis initiation, 78% of the older patients were independent but 1 year later this percentage dropped to 23%. Moreover, within the first 6 months of dialysis treatment, more than 30% of patients had functional loss consequently requiring community or private caregiver support, or to be transfer to a nursing home [18].

Because of the above exposed concepts, the dialysis scheme prescribed to older end-stage renal disease patients should be particularly individualized, taking into account not only their age (old or very old) but also their degree of frailty status (robustness-fragility-terminality). For this reason, four dialysis schemes applicable to the older patient have been proposed based on their functional status and survival prognosis, as follows [45]: conventional dialysis, incremental dialysis, functional dialysis, and palliative dialysis.

1. *Conventional dialysis*: This prescription consists of the standard dialysis scheme, which seeks to achieve a weekly $Kt / V \geq 1.7$ (in the case of PD), and it should be applied to robust oliguric-anuric older patients.
2. *Incremental dialysis*: This prescription consists of a modality that adjusts the dialysis dose in respect to the patient's residual renal function (RRF) in order to achieve an adequate dialysis dose (weekly $Kt / V \geq 1.7$). The incremental dialysis can be applied to robust or vulnerable (pre-fragile) older patients who have a significant volume of residual diuresis. It is worth mentioning that the incremental PD allows older patients to use low dialysate exchange volumes, avoiding the appearance of hernias and/or leakage in this age group. Regarding the incremental HD, this method allows older patients to avoid long dialysis sessions and as a consequence serious complications, such as intradialytic hypotension, arrhythmias, abdominal ischemia, and/or angor.
3. *Functional dialysis*: This prescription consists of a dialysis scheme that manages to provide a minimally useful dialysis dose, although this does not necessarily reach an optimal Kt / V value, but that allows the patient to have acceptable laboratory parameters, as well as maintain his/her clinical functionality, which should be periodically evaluated by validated clinical geriatrics tests (such as walking speed, etc.). In this modality, the residual diuresis (if preserved) is taken into account, and dialysis adequacy parameters other than Kt / V (absence of edema, appetite, uremia values, natremia, serum potassium, etc.) are mainly used to guide the dialysis prescription. Functional dialysis would be applicable to frail older patients whose vital prognosis is not determined by their kidney disease,

but their state of fragility, and have not tolerated conventional or incremental dialytic strategies. In this sense, even though conventional dialysis suggests that anuric patients on PD with daily ultrafiltration ≤750 ml should be monitored and eventually changed to HD, this recommendation does not seem to apply to very old patients, who usually have a low intake of food and fluid, and therefore this cut-off volume value could be excessive in this age subgroup [109–111].

4. *Palliative dialysis*: This prescription consists of a dialytic strategy that only seeks to relieve uremic symptoms and volume overload, without taking into account laboratory parameters or the Kt/V value. Palliative dialysis should be prescribed in a lucid terminal patient, in a state of anuria or oliguria, who has chosen to receive classic palliative treatment without suspending dialysis.

For all these dialysis schemes, the decision of whether to opt for the manual or automated modality depends on the dialysis plan designed by the nephrologist in accordance with the patient's preference. In Fig. 12.1, an algorithm of how each of these dialysis strategies could be applied in the older patient is proposed. However, it should be taken into account that since this algorithm is simply a guideline, it should be reconciled with the patient's will (autonomy) and his/her clinical, family, and social situation (individualized treatment).

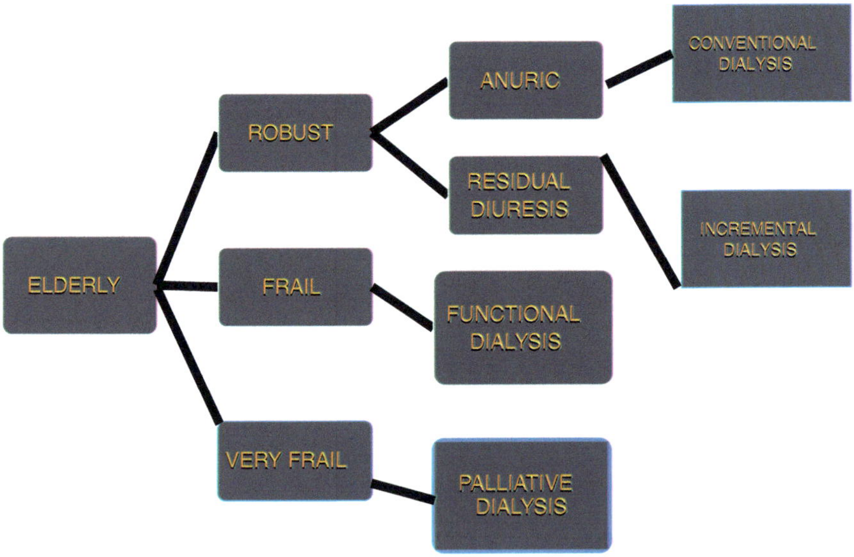

Fig. 12.1 Suggested dialysis prescription algorithm based on frailty evaluation

References

1. Eurostat Statistics Explained. People in the EU – population projections. https://ec.europa.eu/eurostat/statistics-explained/index.php/People_in_the_EU_-_population_projections#Population_projections.
2. Canaud B, Tong L, Tentori F, et al. Clinical practices and outcomes in elderly hemodialysis patients: results from the Dialysis Outcomes and Practice Patterns Study (DOPPS). Clin J Am Soc Nephrol. 2011;6(7):1651–62.
3. Hanafusa N, Nakai S, Iseki K, Tsubakihara Y. Japanese society for dialysis therapy renal data registry—a window through which we can view the details of Japanese dialysis population. Kidney Int Suppl. 2011;5(1):15–22.
4. Saran R, Li Y, Robinson B, Abbott KC, et al. US renal data system 2015 annual data report: epidemiology of kidney disease in the United States. Am J Kidney Dis. 2016;Svii(3 Suppl 1):S1–S305.
5. Nitta K, Hanafusa N, Tsuchiya K. Recent advances in the pathophysiology and management of protein-energy wasting in chronic kidney disease. Ren Replace Ther. 2016;2:4.
6. Roderick PJ. Chronic kidney disease in older people: a cause for concern? Nephrol Dial Transplant. 2011;26(10):3083–6.
7. Musso CG, Trigka K, Dousdampanis P, Jauregui J. Therapeutic alternatives and palliative care for advanced renal disease in the very elderly: a review of the literature. Int Urol Nephrol abril de. 2015;47(4):647–54.
8. Shastri S, Katz R, Rifkin DE, Fried LF, Odden MC, Peralta CA, Chonchol M, Siscovick D, Shlipak MG, Newman AB, Sarnak MJ. Kidney function and mortality in octogenarians: cardiovascular health study all stars. J Am Geriatr Soc. 2012;60(7):1201–7. https://doi.org/10.1111/j.1532-5415.2012.04046.x.
9. Aiello F, Dueñas EP, Musso CG. Senescent nephropathy: the new renal syndrome. Healthcare (Basel). 2017;5(4). pii: E81 https://doi.org/10.3390/healthcare5040081.
10. Rockwood K, Mitnitski A. Frailty defined by deficit accumulation and geriatric medicine defined by frailty. Clin Geriatr Med. 2011;27:17–26.
11. Fried LP, Tangen CM, Walston J, et al. Frailty in older adults: evidence for a phenotype. J Gerontol A Biol Sci Med Sci. 2001;56:M146–56.
12. Wilhelm-Leen ER, Hall YN, Tamura MK, Chertow GM. Frailty and chronic kidney disease: the Third National Health and Nutrition Evaluation Survey. Am J Med. 2009;122(7):664–71.e2.
13. Chowdhury R, Peel NM, Krosch M, Hubbard RE. Frailty and chronic kidney disease: a systematic review. Arch Gerontol Geriatr. 2017;68:135–42.
14. Johansen KL, Chertow GM, Jin C, Kutner NG. Significance of frailty among dialysis patients. J Am Soc Nephrol. 2007;18(11):2960–7.
15. McAdams-DeMarco MA, Law A, Salter ML, et al. Frailty as a novel predictor of mortality and hospitalization in individuals of all ages undergoing hemodialysis. J Am Geriatr Soc. 2013;61:896–901.
16. McAdams-DeMarco MA, Suresh S, Law A, et al. Frailty and falls among adult patients undergoing chronic hemodialysis: a prospective cohort study. BMC Nephrol. 2013;14:224.
17. McAdams-DeMarco MA, Ying H, Olorundare I, et al. Frailty and health-related quality of life in end stage renal disease patients of all ages. J Frailty Aging. 2016;5(3):174–9.
18. Kittiskulnam P, Sheshadri A, Johansen K. Consequences of CKD on functioning. Semin Nephrol. 2016;36(4):305–18. https://doi.org/10.1016/j.semnephrol.2016.05.007.
19. Teitelbaum I. Peritoneal dialysis is appropriate for elderly patients. Contrib Nephrol. 2006; https://doi.org/10.1159/000093600.
20. Johansen KL, Dalrymple LS, Delgado C, et al. Factors associated with frailty and its trajectory among patients on hemodialysis. Clin J Am Soc Nephrol. 2017;12(7):1100–8.
21. Takeuchi H, Uchida HA, Kakio Y. The prevalence of frailty and its associated factors in Japanese hemodialysis patients. Aging Dis. 2018;9(2):192–207.

22. Koopman JJ, Rozing MP, Kramer A, et al. Senescence rates in patients with end-stage renal disease: a critical appraisal of the Gompertz model. Aging Cell. 2011;10(2):233–8.
23. Kim JC, Kalantar-Zadeh K, Kopple JD. Frailty and protein-energy wasting in elderly patients with end stage kidney disease. J Am Soc Nephrol. 2013;24(3):337–51.
24. Johansen KL, Dalrymple LS, Delgado C, et al. Factors associated with frailty and its trajectory among patients on hemodialysis. Clin J Am Soc Nephrol. 2017;12(7):1100–8.
25. Chowdhury R, Peel NM, Krosch M, Hubbard RE. Frailty and chronic kidney disease: a systematic review. Arch Gerontol Geriatr. 2017;68:135–42.
26. Dozio E, Ambrogi F, de Cal M, et al. Role of the soluble Receptor for Advanced Glycation End products (sRAGE) as a prognostic factor for mortality in hemodialysis and peritoneal dialysis patients. Mediat Inflamm. 2018;2018:1347432.
27. Rabbani N, Thornalley PJ. Advanced glycation end products in the pathogenesis of chronic kidney disease. Kidney Int. 2018;93(4):803–13.
28. Bolignano D, Mattace-Raso F, Sijbrands EJ, Zoccali C. The aging kidney revisited: a systematic review. Ageing Res Rev. 2014;14:65–80.
29. Ohashi N, Isobe S, Ishigaki S, et al. Intrarenal renin-angiotensin system activity is augmented after initiation of dialysis. Hypertens Res. 2017;40(4):364–70.
30. Kutner NG, Zhang R, Huang Y, et al. Risk factors for frailty in a large prevalent cohort of hemodialysis patients. Am J Med Sci. 2014;348(4):277–82.
31. Okuyama M, Takeuchi H, Uchida HA, et al. Peripheral artery disease is associated with frailty in chronic hemodialysis patients. Vascular. 2018;26(4):425–31.
32. Kooman JP, Kotanko P, Schols AM, et al. Chronic kidney disease and premature ageing. Nat Rev Nephrol. 2014;10(12):732–42.
33. Valenzuela PL, Cobo F, Diez-Vega I, et al. Physical performance, plasma S-klotho, and all-cause mortality in elderly dialysis patients: a prospective cohort study. Exp Gerontol. 2019;15(122):123–8.
34. Shimoyama Y, Mitsuda Y, Tsuruta Y, et al. SIRTUIN 1 gene polymorphisms are associated with cholesterol metabolism and coronary artery calcification in Japanese hemodialysis patients. J Ren Nutr. 2012;22(1):114–9.
35. McAdams-DeMarco MA, Ying H, Thomas AG, Warsame F, Shaffer AA, Haugen C, Garonzik-Wang JM, Desai NM, Varadhan R, Walston J, Norman SP, Segev DL. Frailty, inflammatory markers, and waitlist mortality among patients with end-stage renal disease in a prospective cohort study. Transplantation. 2018;102(10):1740–6. https://doi.org/10.1097/TP.0000000000002213.
36. Lamarca F, Carrero JJ, Rodrigues JC, et al. Prevalence of sarcopenia in elderly maintenance hemodialysis patients: the impact of different diagnostic criteria. J Nutr Health Aging. 2014;18(7):710–7.
37. Kamijo, Kanda E, Ishibashi Y, Yoshida M. Sarcopenia and frailty in PD: impact on mortality, malnutrition, and inflammation. Perit Dial Int. 2018;38(6):447–54. https://doi.org/10.3747/pdi.2017.00271.
38. Tangvoraphonkchai K, Hung R, Sadeghi-Alavijeh O, Davenport A. Differences in prevalence of muscle weakness (sarcopenia) in haemodialysis patients determined by hand grip strength due to variation in guideline definitions of sarcopenia. Nutr Clin Pract. 2018;33(2):255–60.
39. Malhotra R, Deger SM, Salat H, et al. Sarcopenic obesity definitions by body composition and mortality in the hemodialysis patients. J Ren Nutr. 2017;27(2):84–90.
40. Bataille S, Serveaux M, Carreno E, et al. The diagnosis of sarcopenia is mainly driven by muscle mass in hemodialysis patients. Clin Nutr. 2017;36(6):1654–60.
41. Hara H, Nakamura Y, Hatano M, et al. Protein energy wasting and sarcopenia in dialysis patients. Contrib Nephrol. 2018;196:243–9.
42. Honda H, Qureshi AR, Axelsson J, et al. Obese sarcopenia in patients with end-stage renal disease is associated with inflammation and increased mortality. Am J Clin Nutr. 2007;86(3):633–8.
43. Musso CG, Jauregui JR, Macías Núñez JF. Frailty phenotype and chronic kidney disease: a review of the literature. Int Urol Nephrol. 2015;47(11):1801–7. https://doi.org/10.1007/s11255-015-1112-z.

44. Ostuni M, Musso CG. Usefulness of frailty evaluation for handling chronic kidney disease elderly patients: a review and original proposal. Int Urol Nephrol. 2019;51(3):461–5. https://doi.org/10.1007/s11255-018-2061-0.
45. Musso CG, Trigka K, Dousdampanis P, Jauregui J. Therapeutic alternatives and palliative care for advanced renal disease in the very elderly: a review of the literature. Int Urol Nephrol. 2015;47(4):647–54. https://doi.org/10.1007/s11255-014-0886-8.
46. Johansson L. Nutrition in older adults on peritoneal Dialysis. Perit Dial Int. 2015;35:655–8.
47. Westra WM, Kopple JD, Krediet RT, Appel M, Mehrotra R. Dietary protein requirements and sialysate protein losses in chronic peritoneal dialysis patients. Perit Dial Int. 2007;27:192–5.
48. Santin FG, Bigogno FG, Dias Rodrigues JC, et al. Concurrent and predictive validity of composite methods to assess nutritional status in older adults on hemodialysis. J Ren Nutr. 2016;26(1):18–25.
49. Johansson L, Fouque D, Bellizzi V, et al. European Renal Nutrition (ERN) Working Group of the European Renal Association–European Dialysis Transplant Association (ERA-EDTA). As we grow old: nutritional considerations for older patients on dialysis. Nephrol Dial Transplant. 2017;32(7):1127–36.
50. Sabatino A, Regolisti G, Karupaiah T, et al. Protein-energy wasting and nutritional supplementation in patients with end-stage renal disease on hemodialysis. Clin Nutr. 2017;36(3):663–71.
51. Martins AM, Bello Moreira AS, Canella DS, et al. Elderly patients on hemodialysis have worse dietary quality and higher consumption of ultraprocessed food than elderly without chronic kidney disease. Nutrition. 2017;41:73–9.
52. Sy J, McCulloch CE, Johansen KL. Depressive symptoms, frailty, and mortality among dialysis patients. Hemodial Int. 2019;23(2):239–46.
53. Goto NA, van Loon IN, Morpey MI, et al. Geriatric assessment in elderly patients with end-stage kidney disease. Nephron. 2019;141(1):41–8.
54. Iyasere O, Brown EA, Johansson L, et al. Quality of life with conservative care compared with assisted peritoneal dialysis and haemodialysis. Clin Kidney J. 2018;12(2):262–8.
55. McAdams-DeMarco MA, Tan J, Salter ML, et al. Frailty and cognitive function in incident hemodialysis patients. Clin J Am Soc Nephrol. 2015;10(12):2181–9.
56. van Loon IN, Wouters TR, Boereboom FT, et al. The relevance of geriatric impairments in patients starting Dialysis: a systematic review. Clin J Am Soc Nephrol. 2016;11(7):1245–59.
57. Kallenberg MH, Kleinveld HA, Dekker FW, et al. Functional and cognitive impairment, frailty, and adverse health outcomes in older patients reaching ESRD-A systematic review. Clin J Am Soc Nephrol. 2016;11(9):1624–39.
58. Berkhout-Byrne N, Kallenberg MH, Gaasbeek A, et al. The Cognitive decline in Older Patients with End stage renal disease (COPE) study – rationale and design. Curr Med Res Opin. 2017;33(11):2057–64.
59. Wolfgram DF, Szabo A, Murray AM, Whittle J. Risk of dementia in peritoneal dialysis patients compared with hemodialysis patients. Perit Dial Int. 2015;35(2):189–98.
60. Ali H, Abdelaal F, Baharani J. Assessment of frailty in elderly pre-dialysis population using simple tools. Saudi J Kidney Dis Transpl. 2017;28(4):716–24.
61. Segall L, Nistor I, Van Biesen W, Brown EA, Heaf JG, Lindley E, Farrington K, Covic A. Dialysis modality choice in elderly patients with end-stage renal disease: a narrative review of the available evidence. Nephrol Dial Transplant. 2017;32(1):41–9.
62. Bargman JM. Peritoneal dialysis should be the first choice for renal replacement therapy in the elderly. Semin Dial. 2012; https://doi.org/10.1111/sdi.12013.
63. Brown EA. How to address barriers to peritoneal dialysis in the elderly. Perit Dial Int. 2011;31(Suppl 2):S83–5. https://doi.org/10.3747/pdi.2009.00160.
64. van Loon IN, Joosten H, Iyasere O, et al. The prevalence and impact of falls in elderly dialysis patients: Frail elderly Patient Outcomes on Dialysis (FEPOD) study. Arch Gerontol Geriatr. 2019;83:285–91.
65. Yoneki K, Kitagawa J, Hoshi K, et al. Association between frailty and bone loss in patients undergoing maintenance hemodialysis. J Bone Miner Metab. 2019;37(1):81–9.

66. Cook WL, Tomlinson G, Donaldson M, et al. Falls and fall-related injuries in older dialysis patients. Clin J Am Soc Nephrol. 2006;1(6):1197–204.
67. Cook WL, Jassal SV. Prevalence of falls among seniors maintained on hemodialysis. Int Urol Nephrol. 2005;37(3):649–52.
68. Brown EA. Peritoneal dialysis in the elderly. In: Peritoneal dialysis - from basic concepts to clinical excellence; 2009. https://doi.org/10.1159/000223809.
69. Musso CG, Plazzotta F, Otero C, Aguilera J, Campos F, Diez GR, Luna D, de Quirós FG. Informatic nephrology: 17 years of one-center experience. Int Urol Nephrol. 2015;47(9):1587–8. https://doi.org/10.1007/s11255-015-1060-7.
70. Garcia-Canton C, Rodenas A, Lopez-Aperador C, et al. Frailty in hemodialysis and prediction of poor short-term outcome: mortality, hospitalization and visits to hospital emergency services. Ren Fail. 2019;41(1):567–75.
71. Bowling CB, Hall RK, Khakharia A, et al. Serious fall injury history and adverse health outcomes after initiating hemodialysis among older U.S. adults. J Gerontol A Biol Sci Med Sci. 2018;73(9):1216–21.
72. Kurella Tamura M, Covinsky KE, Chertow GM, et al. Functional status of elderly adults before and after initiation of dialysis. N Engl J Med. 2009;361(16):1539–47.
73. Couchoud CG, Beuscart JB, Aldigier JC, et al. REIN registry: development of a risk stratification algorithm to improve patient-centered care and decision making for incident elderly patients with end-stage renal disease. Kidney Int. 2005;88:1178–86.
74. Sclauzero P, Galli G, Barbati G, et al. Role of components of frailty on quality of life in dialysis patients: a cross-sectional study. J Ren Care. 2013;39(2):96–102.
75. Iyasere OU, Brown EA, Johansson L, et al. Quality of life and physical function in older patients on dialysis: a comparison of assisted peritoneal Dialysis with hemodialysis. Clin J Am Soc Nephrol. 2016;11(3):423–30.
76. Genestier S, Meyer N, Chantrel F, Alenabi F, Brignon P, Maaz M, Muller S, Faller B. Prognostic survival factors in elderly renal failure patients treated with peritoneal Dialysis: a nine-year retrospective study. Perit Dial Int. J Int Soc Perit Dial. 2010;30(2):218–26.
77. Iyasere OU, Brown EA, Johansson L, Huson L, Smee J, Maxwell AP, Farrington K, Davenport A. Quality of life and physical function in older patients on dialysis: a comparison of assisted peritoneal dialysis with hemodialysis. Clin J Am Soc Nephrol. 2016;11(3):423–30.
78. Nitta K, Hanafusa N, Tsuchiya K. Role of frailty on outcomes of dialysis patients. Contrib Nephrol. 2018;195:102–9.
79. Brown EA, Farrington K. Geriatric assessment in advanced kidney disease. Clin J Am Soc Nephrol. 2019;14(7):1091–3.
80. Ellis G, Whitehead MA, Robinson D, et al. Comprehensive geriatric assessment for older adults admitted to hospital: meta-analysis of randomized controlled trials. BMJ. 2011;343:d6553.
81. Parlevliet JL, Buurman BM, Pannekeet MMH, et al. Systematic comprehensive geriatric assessment in elderly patients on chronic dialysis: a cross-sectional comparative and feasibility study. BMC Nephrol. 2012;13:30.
82. Hall RK, Haines C, Gorbatkin SM, et al. Incorporating geriatric assessment into a nephrology clinic: preliminary data from two models of care. J Am Geriatr Soc. 2016;64:2154–8.
83. Wiggins J, Bitzer M. Geriatric assessment for the nephrologist. Semin Dial. 2012;25:623–7.
84. Ramer SJ, McCall NN, Robinson-Cohen C, et al. Health outcome priorities of older adults with advanced CKD and concordance with their nephrology providers' perceptions. J Am Soc Nephrol. 2018;29:2870–8.
85. Carrero JJ, Stenvinkel P, Cuppari L, et al. Etiology of the protein-energy wasting syndrome in chronic kidney disease: a consensus statement from the International Society of Renal Nutrition and Metabolism (ISRNM). J Ren Nutr. 2013;23:77–90.
86. Villain C, Ecochard R, Bouchet J-L, et al. Relative prognostic impact of nutrition, anaemia, bone metabolism and cardiovascular comorbidities in elderly haemodialysis patients. Nephrol Dial Transplant. 2019;34(5):848–58.
87. Farrington K, Covic A, Aucella F, et al. Clinical practice guideline on management of older patients with chronic kidney disease stage 3b or higher (eGFR <45 mL/min/1.73 m^2). Nephrol Dial Transplant. 2016;31(Suppl 2):ii1–ii66.

88. Ritter CS, Slatopolsky E. Phosphate toxicity in CKD: the killer among us. Clin J Am Soc Nephrol. 2016;11:1088–100.
89. Kopple JD. The National Kidney Foundation K/DOQI clinical practice guidelines for dietary protein intake for chronic dialysis patients. Am J Kidney Dis. 2001;38(4 Suppl 1):S68–73.
90. Toigo G, Aparicio M, Attman P-O, et al. Expert working group report on nutrition in adult patients with renal insufficiency (part 2 of 2). Clin Nutr. 2000;19:281–91.
91. Naylor HL, Jackson H, Walker GH, et al. British Dietetic Association evidence-based guidelines for the protein requirements of adults undergoing maintenance haemodialysis or peritoneal dialysis. J Hum Nutr Diet. 2013;26:315–28.
92. Fouque D, Vennegoor M, Ter Wee P, et al. EBPG guideline on nutrition. Nephrol Dial Transplant. 2007;22(Suppl 2):ii45–87.
93. Ikizler TA, Cano NJ, Franch H, et al. Prevention and treatment of protein energy wasting in chronic kidney disease patients: a consensus statement by the International Society of Renal Nutrition and Metabolism. Kidney Int. 2013;84:1096–107.
94. Johansen KL, Painter P, Kent-Braun JA, et al. Validation of questionnaires to estimate physical activity and functioning in end-stage renal disease. Kidney Int. 2001;59:1121–7.
95. Johansen KL, Kaysen GA, Dalrymple LS, et al. Association of physical activity with survival among ambulatory patients on dialysis: the comprehensive dialysis study. Clin J Am Soc Nephrol. 2013;8:248–53.
96. Johansen KL. Exercise in the end-stage renal disease population. J Am Soc Nephrol. 2007;18:1845–54.
97. Painter PL. Exercise in end-stage renal disease. Exerc Sport Sci Rev. 1988;16:305–39.
98. Tentori F, Elder SJ, Thumma J, et al. Physical exercise among participants in the Dialysis Outcomes and Practice Patterns Study (DOPPS): correlates and associated outcomes. Nephrol Dial Transplant. 2010;25(9):3050–62.
99. Hristea D, Deschamps T, Paris A, et al. Combining intra-dialytic exercise and nutritional supplementation in malnourished older haemodialysis patients: towards better quality of life and autonomy. Nephrology (Carlton). 2016;21(9):785–90.
100. Manfredini F, Mallamaci F, D'Arrigo G, et al. Exercise in patients on dialysis: a multicenter, randomized clinical trial. J Am Soc Nephrol. 2017;28:1259–68.
101. Boston Working Group on Improving Health Care. Outcomes through geriatric rehabilitation. Med Care. 1997;35:JS4–JS20.
102. Farragher J, Jassal SV. Rehabilitation of the geriatric dialysis patient. Semin Dial. 2012;25(6):649–56.
103. Li M, Porter E, Lam R, Jassal S. Quality improvement through the introduction of interdisciplinary geriatric hemodialysis rehabilitation care. Am J Kidney Dis. 2007;50:90–7.
104. Heung M, Adamowski T, Segal JH, Malani PN. A successful approach to fall prevention in an outpatient hemodialysis center. Clin J Am Soc Nephrol. 2010;5:1775–9.
105. Ortiz A, Sanchez-niño M. Sarcopenia in CKD: a roadmap from basic pathogenetic mechanisms to clinical trials. Clin Kidney J. 2019;12(1):110–2.
106. Nessim SJ, Bargman JM, Austin PC, Story K, Jassal SV. Impact of age on peritonitis risk in peritoneal dialysis patients: an era effect. Clin J Am Soc Nephrol. 2009;4(1):135–41.
107. Lim WH, Dogra GK, McDonald SF, Brown FG, Johnson DW. Compared with younger peritoneal dialysis patients, elderly patients have similar peritonitis-free survival and lower risk of technique failure, but higher risk of peritonitis-related mortality. Perit Dial Int. 2011;31:663–71.
108. Capotondo MM, Musso CG. Nephroprevention in the elderly. In: Musso CG, Jauregui JR, Macías-Núñez JF, Covic A, editors. . Cham: Springer; 2019.
109. Musso CG, Schwartz P, Deira J, Macias Núñez JF. Is it correct to use a unique conventional dialysis prescription in the elderly? Four alternative schedules for dialyzing elderly patients. Int J Ren Dis Ther. 2018;1(1):103.
110. Oei E, Fan S. Peritoneal dialysis adequacy in elderly patients. Perit Dial Int J Int Soc Perit Dial. 2015;35(6):635–9.
111. Htay H, Cho Y, Pascoe EM, Darssan D, Nadeau-Fredette A-C, Hawley C, Clayton PA, et al. Multicenter registry analysis of center characteristics associated with technique failure in patients on incident peritoneal dialysis. Clin J Am Soc Nephrol. 2017;12(7):1090–9.

Chapter 13
Frailty in Kidney Transplantation

Candela Conti, Dana M. Mysler, Gabriel Echeverri, and Kristian Heldal

Introduction

Age per se is an unreliable marker of senescence (pathological aging), and consequently, frailty status assessment has become a crucial marker for distinguishing between normal aging and senescence [1, 2]. Frailty is a syndrome characterized by the inability of the organism to respond efficiently to stressors (reduced homeostasis) and represents a chronic inflammatory status which leads to an altered immune response, neuroendocrine changes, and cognitive impairment [1, 3–14].

Kidney transplantation (KT) is regarded as the optimal alternative treatment for end-stage renal disease (ESRD) patients [3, 14, 15], and among the recognized factors related to renal graft deterioration, is the graft senescence itself [16, 17]. KT recovery is potentially challenging for vulnerable recipients, since during this period, recipients are at high risk of complications following acute rejection episodes in addition to postsurgical complications [14, 15, 18, 19].

KT patients who are classified as frail (young or old) seem to have higher risk of developing graft inflammation, a situation that can lead to poor outcomes. Moreover, frailty could lead to adverse health outcomes through behavioral and medical care changes affected by poor cognitive function [20].

Therefore, determining the severity of frailty in KT candidates and recipients can help physicians to better address decision-making in this population [1–14, 20–24].

C. Conti · D. M. Mysler
Physiology Department, Instituto Universitario del Hospital Italiano de Buenos Aires, Buenos Aires, Argentina

G. Echeverri
Clinica de la Costa, Barranquilla, Colombia

K. Heldal (✉)
Department of Transplantation Medicine, Section of Nephrology, Oslo University Hospital, Oslo, Norway
e-mail: hkri@ous-hf.no

© Springer Nature Switzerland AG 2021

C. G. Musso et al. (eds.), *Frailty and Kidney Disease*,
https://doi.org/10.1007/978-3-030-53529-2_13

Waitlist and Frailty

It is well documented that the waitlist mortality is almost twice as high among frail KT candidates compared with their robust peers. At 3 years on the waiting list, the cumulative mortality rate was 18% versus 10%, and at 5 years the cumulative mortality rate had increased to 33% versus 18% [4]. In addition, an association between frailty, markers of inflammation, and mortality has been documented, showing that inflammation markers, particularly IL-6, improve mortality risk prediction among ESRD patients on the KT waitlist [1, 8, 12, 25, 26].

KT is associated with better survival relative to dialysis even among high-risk subgroups (e.g., older, etc.) [27–29]. However, transplant centers may preferentially select the most resilient candidates for waitlisting, since individuals with physical or cognitive impairment are thought to suffer from more complications after transplant surgery and immunosuppression and also have a higher risk of medication nonadherence [3].

Frail patients are less likely to be listed for kidney transplantation, and they have also been shown to have higher waitlist mortality and consequently lower transplant rate compared to non-frail patients [4, 18]. This phenomenon could be explained by the longer time to evaluate frail patients for transplantation, their higher degree of comorbidities, higher age, and longer waiting time for deceased kidney transplantation [18].

It is though important to remember that frailty is a potentially modifiable risk factor and that improvement of frailty status through prehabilitation may increase patient access to KT and thereby improve their outcomes [4, 18, 22, 30].

Kidney Transplantation Frail Patients

Both normal aging and senescence affect the immune response, a phenomenon which can be related to higher rates of infections and malignancies with increasing age. In normal aging, the pro-inflammatory cytokine IL-6 has been detected at very low levels, while high levels of IL-6 have been associated with senescence and with several chronic diseases associated to aging. Specific immune changes are characteristic for frailty, such as higher amounts of CD8+ cells and CD8+ CD28− lymphocytes and a lower CD4+:CD8+ ratio compared to robust older individuals. Moreover, frail patients often show increased numbers of T cells which express the chemokine CCR5, a chemokine receptor which correlates with the frailty degree. Increased inflammatory cytokine levels in frail patients have been associated with delayed graft function (DGF) in KT [1].

Frailty is found in up to 20% of KT recipients of all ages, and it has been associated with an increased risk of adverse postoperative outcomes: delirium, delayed graft function (DGF), increased length of hospital stay, early hospital readmission, mycophenolate mofetil (MMF) intolerance, and higher mortality [1, 3–5, 20–22, 31].

Both frailty and DGF have been linked to a pro-inflammatory state associated with overexpression of several inflammatory cytokines. The risk of DGF has been found to be twice as high in frail KT recipients compared to their robust peers [13, 14, 32]. Moreover, frailty has been identified as a robust predictor of 30-day postoperative complications independent of age [1, 3–5, 20–22, 31].

Studies have reported that even patients with limited functional status may live longer with KT compared to dialysis, and it is likely that many frail and cognitively impaired patients would also live longer if they were transplanted. Future studies should investigate whether prehabilitation of frail patients will improve the outcomes after transplantation and also evaluate if it is possible to improve adherence by use of directed support to some patients. The most important contribution to improvement of outcomes will however be an introduction of a reliable tool with a defined cutoff value that can be used in selection of patients ensuring that each patient is provided the best treatment option [3, 4].

Kidney Transplantation Frail Patients: Frailty Evaluation

Since functional deterioration is gradual, frailty trends could be identified by analyzing trajectory curves similar to growth curves used by pediatricians. In early stages of frailty, patients may benefit from an intervention aiming to improve the patient's frailty status (window opportunity), while rehabilitation may not be efficient among patients with higher degree of frailty [3]. Staging of frailty could consequently serve as an important tool in the decision of when to prescribe physical rehabilitation to try to turn a vulnerable (pre-frail) patient into a robust one.

Frailty staging is usually performed by using the following alternative categorizations [30, 33–36]:

(a) Binary score: frail or robust
(b) Tertiary score: frail, intermediately frail, or robust

In a recent study, Chu et al. found that among KT candidates who were categorized by applying the binary frailty score classification, 7% remained frail, 74% remained robust, 10% transitioned from frail to robust, and 9% transitioned from robust to frail, while among KT candidates who were categorized by applying the tertiary frailty score classification, 22% became frailer, 25% became less frail, and 7% remained frail, 10% intermediate frail, and 36% robust. In addition, with each year on dialysis, candidates were less likely to transition from frail to robust, and patients with diabetes mellitus had a higher risk of remaining frail. For three-category frailty score, those candidates who became more frail between evaluation and KT had a 2.27-fold higher risk of post-KT mortality compared to individuals who remained stable. Besides, among patients who had increased frailty score, the risk of mortality was 2.36-fold higher than for those who remained stable. Therefore, this study demonstrated that frailty is a subject to change while KT candidates are on the waitlist. Thus, KT candidates became more or less frail between evaluation and KT regardless of the frailty score used, and consequently serial measurements of frailty may be justified while patients are on the waiting list [5].

The cognitive function of transplant candidates has been studied by applying the Montreal Cognitive Assessment (MoCA), a brief 30-question cognitive test developed for evaluation of dementia. KT candidates with low MoCA had longer median time to listing than those with higher scores, but this association was attenuated after multivariable adjustment [3, 20].

Regarding frailty evaluation after kidney transplantation, it is documented that independent of recipient age, with increasing time after KT, the proportion of KT recipients who were less frail increased, whereas the proportion of patients who were more frail than at the time of KT was reduced. Frailty scores were initially worsened after KT, but already at 3 months after KT, the scores were better than they were at the time of KT. It has been proposed that frailty initially worsened, because of the surgical procedure and immunosuppressive treatment, but then improved, presumably because of the restoration of renal function, supporting transplantation in these individuals and suggesting that pretransplantation frailty is not an irreversible status [15].

It is worth mentioning that KT frail recipients are usually older compared to robust recipients, and they are more likely than robust KT recipients to present with depression, disabilities, and poor HRQOL. However, the proportion of KT frail recipients who experienced rejection within 1 year posttransplant does not differ from that of robust recipients [20].

Kidney Transplantation Frail Patients: Clinical Characteristics

Studies using the Fried frailty phenotype indicate that frail and vulnerable patients with ESRD and solid organ transplant recipients have inferior clinical outcomes [37–39]. The most common comorbidities, such as diabetes mellitus and congestive heart failure, have synergistic effect of the frailty burden. However, in frail wait-listed patients, frailty by itself is considered to be a greater risk factor for mortality than other comorbid conditions [21].

Cognitive impairment is highly prevalent among older patients with CKD, and the prevalence of cognitive decline in ESRD varies between 16% and 38%. Besides, chronic inflammation, anemia, and hypertension related to ESRD have all been associated with development of cognitive dysfunction. In this sense, it has been documented that both frail and robust kidney graft recipients experienced short-term improvements in cognitive function posttransplantation [1]. However, between 1 and 4 years posttransplant, robust recipients maintained higher levels of cognitive function, while frail recipients experienced cognitive decline [20].

It has been reported that about 10% of KT recipients had depression, 16% were frail, and 4% exhibited both frailty and depressive symptoms. Depressive patients had a 3.97-fold higher likelihood of suffering from frailty phenotype. Moreover, KT frail recipients who suffered from depression experience a 6.20-fold increased risk of DGF and a 2.62-fold increased risk of mortality, compared to robust KT recipients without depression [6]. However, the synergistic effect of frailty and depressive symptoms only impacted short-term outcomes, but did not have a synergistic long-term effect [6].

Early hospital readmission (EHR), defined as rehospitalization within 30 days of initial post-KT discharge, has been associated with avoidable morbidity, increased cost, and transition of care problems. EHR has become a significant metric for hospital quality. Almost one-third of KT recipients are readmitted to the hospital within 30 days of discharge. Researchers found that frailty was independently associated with EHR, and did not differ based on age or ethnicity [32, 40]. Additionally, polypharmacy has been identified as a risk factor for adverse drug reactions and unplanned hospital readmission, and frailty has been linked to a higher risk of adverse drug reactions. Therefore, if frail patients are approved for KT, a polypharmacy reduction may be beneficial [1].

Kidney Transplantation Frail Patients: Health-Related Quality of Life

Health-related quality of life (HRQOL) is an important marker of patient's disease burden and treatment effectiveness. Poor HRQOL is associated with increased risks of hospitalizations, graft failure, and mortality in KT patients. It has been demonstrated that frail ESRD patients are more than twice as likely to experience a decline in HRQOL while awaiting KT, resulting in worse HRQOL compared to robust peers. Moreover, particular entities, such as sarcopenia and diabetes mellitus, are characteristically associated with worse physical HRQOL after KT. However, KT frail recipients had worse physical and kidney disease-specific HRQOL prior to KT, but they had a greater rate of improvement in the first 3 months post-KT compared with their robust peers. It is possible that while KT frail recipients experience the greatest decline in HRQOL while undergoing the stressor of dialysis, renal function restoration through KT improved their HRQOL even if they experienced EHR or DGF. Conversely, there were no differences in mental HRQOL or changes in mental HRQOL at KT by frailty status [41]. These findings highlight that even a high-risk group like KT frail recipients can experience the benefit of improved HRQOL with KT [41, 42].

Kidney Transplantation Frail Patients: Physical Performance and Sarcopenia

Frailty and physical performance have been shown to be independently associated with increased mortality after KT [18]. Physical performance can be investigated by standardized, objective tools as the short physical performance battery (SPPB) [43].

Standardized measurement of psoas muscle volume in CT scans as an expression of sarcopenia has been described to be an independent predictor of mortality and major morbidity after heart, lung, and liver transplantation [44–46]. A similar association has to our knowledge so far not been described in KT, but it is reasonable to believe that it also exists in this population. Since an abdominal CT scan is often used as a regular part of the evaluation of KT candidates, it would be feasible if one could use automated measurements of psoas muscle volume in the risk stratification process.

Kidney Transplantation Frail Patients: Therapeutic Particularities

Immunosuppression after KT represents a major stressor to recipients, and it is possible that KT frail patients do not have the resiliency to withstand standard doses of immunosuppressants and consequently require a dose reduction or discontinuation. However, those patients who require a dose reduction are at increased risk of acute rejection and graft loss [11]. Acute rejection has also been found to be associated with increased mortality in KT recipients older than 70 years [19]. The prevalence of MMF dose reduction was 1.3 times greater for those patients who were classified as frail compared to those who were robust. This association between frailty and MMF dose reduction was neither modified by age, donor type, sex, nor race [11].

Regarding frailty treatment, multiple interventions have been proposed (e.g., exercise training, hormonal replacement, etc.) to increase maximal oxygen uptake and improve muscle strength in frail older individuals. Several studies have demonstrated improved gait speed, balance, and functional outcomes with structured physical activity programs. In addition, improving nutrition represents an additional supportive treatment approach, and studies have shown a beneficial effect on the progress of sarcopenia with an augmented protein intake, while applying nutritional guidelines and nutritional supplements may represent helpful interventions in frail patients before surgery [1, 47].

Conclusion

Even though KT frail recipients are high-risk candidates compared to robust peers, they can improve their frailty status with prehabilitation before surgery and thereby also improve their clinical outcomes after transplantation. Therefore, frailty assessment should be performed in KT candidates for their optimal medical assistance. Future research should aim to establish cutoff values for frailty scores that can be implemented in the selection criteria for KT ensuring that the individual patient receives the best available treatment and that donor organs are utilized in an optimal way.

References

1. Exterkate L, Slegtenhorst BR, Kelm M, Seyda M, Schuitenmaker JM, Quante M, Uehara H, El Khal A, Tullius SG. Frailty and transplantation. Transplantation. 2016;100(4):727–33. https://doi.org/10.1097/TP.0000000000001003.
2. Aiello F, Dueñas EP, Musso CG. Senescent nephropathy: the new renal syndrome. Healthcare (Basel). 2017;5(4):E81. https://doi.org/10.3390/healthcare5040081.
3. Harhay MN, Reese PP. Frailty and cognitive deficits limit access to kidney transplantation: unfair or unavoidable? Clin J Am Soc Nephrol. 2019;14(4):493–5. https://doi.org/10.2215/CJN.02390219.
4. Haugen CE, Chu NM, Ying H, Warsame F, Holscher CM, Desai NM, Jones MR, Norman SP, Brennan DC, Garonzik-Wang J, Walston JD, Bingaman AW, Segev DL, McAdams-DeMarco M. Frailty and access to kidney transplantation. Clin J Am Soc Nephrol. 2019;14(4):576–82. https://doi.org/10.2215/CJN.12921118.
5. Chu NM, Deng A, Ying H, Haugen CE, Garonzik Wang JM, Segev DL, McAdams-DeMarco MA. Dynamic frailty before kidney transplantation: time of measurement matters. Transplantation. 2019;103(8):1700–4. https://doi.org/10.1097/TP.0000000000002563.
6. Konel JM, Warsame F, Ying H, Haugen CE, Mountford A, Chu NM, Crews DC, Desai NM, Garonzik-Wang JM, Walston JD, Norman SP, Segev DL, McAdams-DeMarco MA. Depressive symptoms, frailty, and adverse outcomes among kidney transplant recipients. Clin Transpl. 2018;32(10):e13391. https://doi.org/10.1111/ctr.13391.
7. Schopmeyer L, El Moumni M, Nieuwenhuijs-Moeke GJ, Berger SP, Bakker SJL, Pol RA. Frailty has a significant influence on postoperative complications after kidney transplantation-a prospective study on short-term outcomes. Transpl Int. 2019;32(1):66–74. https://doi.org/10.1111/tri.13330.
8. McAdams-DeMarco MA, Ying H, Thomas AG, Warsame F, Shaffer AA, Haugen CE, Garonzik-Wang JM, Desai NM, Varadhan R, Walston J, Norman SP, Segev DL. Frailty, inflammatory markers, and waitlist mortality among patients with end-stage renal disease in a prospective cohort study. Transplantation. 2018;102(10):1740–6. https://doi.org/10.1097/TP.0000000000002213.
9. Brett KE, Bennett A, Ritchie LJ, Knoll GA. Physical frailty and functional status in patients with advanced kidney disease: a protocol for a systematic review. Syst Rev. 2017;6(1):133. https://doi.org/10.1186/s13643-017-0536-1.
10. Alfaadhel TA, Soroka SD, Kiberd BA, Landry D, Moorhouse P, Tennankore KK. Frailty and mortality in dialysis: evaluation of a clinical frailty scale. Clin J Am Soc Nephrol. 2015;10(5):832–40. https://doi.org/10.2215/CJN.07760814.
11. McAdams-DeMarco MA, Law A, Tan J, Delp C, King EA, Orandi B, Salter M, Alachkar N, Desai N, Grams M, Walston J, Segev DL. Frailty, mycophenolate reduction, and graft loss in kidney transplant recipients. Transplantation. 2015;99(4):805–10. https://doi.org/10.1097/TP.0000000000000444.
12. McAdams-DeMarco MA, Law A, King E, Orandi B, Salter M, Gupta N, Chow E, Alachkar N, Desai N, Varadhan R, Walston J, Segev DL. Frailty and mortality in kidney transplant recipients. Am J Transplant. 2015;15(1):149–54. https://doi.org/10.1111/ajt.12992.
13. No authors listed. Simple "frailty" test predicts kidney transplant outcome:gauge of physical reserve not just for elderly. Home Healthc Nurse. 2012;30(6):328–30. https://doi.org/10.1097/NHH.0b013e3182575465.
14. Garonzik-Wang JM, Govindan P, Grinnan JW, Liu M, Ali HM, Chakraborty A, Jain V, Ros RL, James NT, Kucirka LM, Hall EC, Berger JC, Montgomery RA, Desai NM, Dagher NN, Sonnenday CJ, Englesbe MJ, Makary MA, Walston JD, Segev DL. Frailty and delayed graft function in kidney transplant recipients. Arch Surg. 2012;147(2):190–3. https://doi.org/10.1001/archsurg.2011.1229.

15. McAdams-DeMarco MA, Isaacs K, Darko L, Salter ML, Gupta N, King EA, Walston J, Segev DL. Changes in frailty after kidney transplantation. J Am Geriatr Soc. 2015;63(10):2152–7. https://doi.org/10.1111/jgs.13657.
16. Musso CG, Giordani MC, Imperiali N. Aging kidney transplantation. Rev Investig Clin. 2016;68(2):68–74.
17. Musso CG, Heldal K. How to differentiate kidney graft ageing from kidney graft progeria: a simple and practical proposal. Electron J Biomed. 2017;2:3–5.
18. Lorenz EC, Cosio FG, Bernard SL, Bogard SD, Bjerke BR, Geissler EN, Hanna SW, Kremers WK, Cheng Y, Stegall MD, Cheville AL, LeBrasseur NK. The relationship between frailty and decreased physical performance with death on the kidney transplant waiting list. Prog Transplant. 2019;29(2):108–14. https://doi.org/10.1177/1526924819835803.
19. Heldal K, Hartmann A, Leivestad T, Svendsen MV, Foss A, Lien B, Midtvedt K. Clinical outcomes in elderly kidney transplant recipients are related to acute rejection episodes rather than pretransplant comorbidity. Transplantation. 2009;87(7):1045–51. https://doi.org/10.1097/TP.0b013e31819cdddd.
20. Chu NM, Gross AL, Shaffer AA, Haugen CE, Norman SP, Xue QL, Sharrett AR, Carlson MC, Bandeen-Roche K, Segev DL, McAdams-DeMarco MA. Frailty and changes in cognitive function after kidney transplantation. J Am Soc Nephrol. 2019;30(2):336–45. https://doi.org/10.1681/ASN.2018070726.
21. Pérez Fernández M, Martínez Miguel P, Ying H, Haugen CE, Chu NM, Rodríguez Puyol DM, Rodríguez-Mañas L, Norman SP, Walston JD, Segev DL, McAdams-DeMarco MA. Comorbidity, frailty, and waitlist mortality among kidney transplant candidates of all ages. Am J Nephrol. 2019;49(2):103–10. https://doi.org/10.1159/000496061.
22. Kobashigawa J, Dadhania D, Bhorade S, Adey D, Berger J, Bhat G, Budev M, Duarte-Rojo A, Dunn M, Hall S, Harhay MN, Johansen KL, Joseph S, Kennedy CC, Kransdorf E, Lentine KL, Lynch RJ, McAdams-DeMarco M, Nagai S, Olymbios M, Patel J, Pinney S, Schaenman J, Segev DL, Shah P, Singer LG, Singer JP, Sonnenday C, Tandon P, Tapper E, Tullius SG, Wilson M, Zamora M, Lai JC. Report from the American Society of Transplantation on frailty in solid organ transplantation. Am J Transplant. 2019;19(4):984–94. https://doi.org/10.1111/ajt.15198.
23. Brown EA, Johansson L. Old age and frailty in the dialysis population. J Nephrol. 2010;23(5):502–7.
24. Musso CG, Vilas M, de Quirós FG, Núñez JF. The importance of evaluating frailty and social-behavioral factors for managing drugs and dialysis prescription in elderly patients. Drug Res (Stuttg). 2016;66(4):223–4. https://doi.org/10.1055/s-0035-1565127.
25. Chowdhury R, Peel NM, Krosch M, Hubbard RE. Frailty and chronic kidney disease: a systematic review. Arch Gerontol Geriatr. 2017;68:135–42. https://doi.org/10.1016/j.archger.2016.10.007.
26. Pugh J, Aggett J, Goodland A, Prichard A, Thomas N, Donovan K, Roberts G. Frailty and comorbidity are independent predictors of outcome in patients referred for pre-dialysis education. Clin Kidney J. 2016;9(2):324–9. https://doi.org/10.1093/ckj/sfv150.
27. Wolfe RA, Ashby VB, Milford EL, Ojo AO, Ettenger RE, Agodoa LY, Held PJ, Port FK. Comparison of mortality in all patients on dialysis, patients on dialysis awaiting transplantation, and recipients of a first cadaveric transplant. N Engl J Med. 1999;341(23):1725–30.
28. Rao PS, Schaubel DE, Jia X, Li S, Port FK, Saran R. Survival on dialysis post-kidney transplant failure: results from the Scientific Registry of Transplant Recipients. Am J Kidney Dis. 2007;49(2):294–300.
29. Heldal K, Hartmann A, Grootendorst DC, de Jager DJ, Leivestad T, Foss A, Midtvedt K. Benefit of kidney transplantation beyond 70 years of age. Nephrol Dial Transplant. 2010;25(5):1680–7. https://doi.org/10.1093/ndt/gfp681.
30. Feng S, Nie L, Wolfe RA. Laplace's approximation for relative risk frailty models. Lifetime Data Anal. 2009;15(3):343–56. https://doi.org/10.1007/s10985-009-9112-x.
31. Goldfarb DA. Re: frailty and mortality in kidney transplant recipients. J Urol. 2015;194(2):483. https://doi.org/10.1016/j.juro.2015.03.016.

32. McAdams-DeMarco MA, Law A, Salter ML, Chow E, Grams M, Walston J, Segev DL. Frailty and early hospital readmission after kidney transplantation. Am J Transplant. 2013;13(8):2091–5. https://doi.org/10.1111/ajt.12300.
33. Liu L, Wolfe RA, Huang X. Shared frailty models for recurrent events and a terminal event. Biometrics. 2004;60(3):747–56.
34. Sieverdes JC, Rao V, Taber DJ, Noltemeyer Z, McGillicuddy JW, Bergamin M, Thangavel S, Baliga PK. Feasibility and functional testing for frailty in chronic kidney disease. Prog Transplant. 2018;28(3):299–300. https://doi.org/10.1177/1526924818781577.
35. Van Pilsum Rasmussen S, Konel J, Warsame F, Ying H, Buta B, Haugen C, King E, DiBrito S, Varadhan R, Rodríguez-Mañas L, Walston JD, Segev DL, McAdams-DeMarco MA. Engaging clinicians and patients to assess and improve frailty measurement in adults with end stage renal disease. BMC Nephrol. 2018;19(1):8. https://doi.org/10.1186/s12882-017-0806-0.
36. Adlam T, Ulrich E, Kent M, Malinzak L. Frailty testing pilot study: pros and pitfalls. J Clin Med Res. 2018;10(2):82–7. https://doi.org/10.14740/jocmr3203w.
37. Mauthner O, Claes V, Walston J, Engberg S, Binet I, Dickenmann M5, Golshayan D, Hadaya K, Huynh-Do U, Calciolari S, De Geest S, GERAS study consortium; For the Psychosocial Interest Group; Swiss Transplant Cohort Study (STCS). ExplorinG frailty and mild cognitive impairmEnt in kidney tRansplantation to predict biomedicAl, psychosocial and health cost outcomeS (GERAS): protocol of a nationwide prospective cohort study. J Adv Nurs. 2017;73(3):716–34. https://doi.org/10.1111/jan.13179.
38. McAdams-DeMarco MA, Ying H, Olorundare I, King EA, Haugen C, Buta B, Gross AL, Kalyani R, Desai NM, Dagher NN, Lonze BE, Montgomery RA, Bandeen-Roche K, Walston JD, Segev DL. Individual frailty components and mortality in kidney transplant recipients. Transplantation. 2017;101(9):2126–32. https://doi.org/10.1097/TP.0000000000001546.
39. McAdams-DeMarco MA, King EA, Luo X, Haugen C, DiBrito S, Shaffer A, Kucirka LM, Desai NM, Dagher NN, Lonze BE, Montgomery RA, Walston J, Segev DL. Frailty, length of stay, and mortality in kidney transplant recipients: a National Registry and Prospective Cohort Study. Ann Surg. 2017;266(6):1084–90. https://doi.org/10.1097/SLA.0000000000002025.
40. Goldfarb DA. Re: frailty and early hospital readmission after kidney transplantation. J Urol. 2014;191(5):1366. https://doi.org/10.1016/j.juro.2014.02.016.
41. McAdams-DeMarco MA, Olorundare IO, Ying H, Warsame F, Haugen CE, Hall R, Garonzik-Wang JM, Desai NM, Walston JD, Norman SP, Segev DL. Frailty and postkidney transplant health-related quality of life. Transplantation. 2018;102(2):291–9. https://doi.org/10.1097/TP.0000000000001943.
42. McAdams-DeMarco MA, Ying H, Olorundare I, King EA, Desai N, Dagher N, Lonze B, Montgomery R, Walston J, Segev DL. Frailty and health-related quality of life in end stage renal disease patients of all ages. J Frailty Aging. 2016;5(3):174–9.
43. Guralnik JM, Simonsick EM, Ferrucci L, Glynn RJ, Berkman LF, Blazer DG, Scherr PA, Wallace RB. A short physical performance battery assessing lower extremity function: association with self-reported disability and prediction of mortality and nursing home admission. J Gerontol. 1994;49(2):M85–94.
44. Bibas L, Saleh E, Al-Kharji S, Chetrit J, Mullie L, Cantarovich M, Cecere R, Giannetti N, Afilalo J. Muscle mass and mortality after cardiac transplantation. Transplantation. 2018;102(12):2101–7. https://doi.org/10.1097/TP.0000000000002311.
45. Hsu J, Krishnan A, Lin CT, Shah PD, Broderick SR, Higgins RSD, Merlo CA, Bush EL. Sarcopenia of the psoas muscles is associated with poor outcomes following lung transplantation. Ann Thorac Surg. 2019;107(4):1082–8. https://doi.org/10.1016/j.athoracsur.2018.10.006.
46. Izumi T, Watanabe J, Tohyama T, Takada Y. Impact of psoas muscle index on short-term outcome after living donor liver transplantation. Turk J Gastroenterol. 2016;27(4):382–8. https://doi.org/10.5152/tjg.2016.16201.
47. Musso CG, Jauregui JR, Macías Núñez JF. Frailty phenotype and chronic kidney disease: a review of the literature. Int Urol Nephrol. 2015;47(11):1801–7. https://doi.org/10.1007/s11255-015-1112-z.

Chapter 14
Chronic Kidney Disease Continuous Care (Supportive and Conservative Treatment)

Carlos Zuñiga-San Martin

Introduction

Chronic kidney disease (CKD) is a public health problem that is increasing in prevalence and incidence worldwide [1–8]. The prevalence is currently estimated at 11% and 13% of the world's general population [9] which is variable according to socioeconomic level and ethnicity among other health determinants [10].

Early diagnosis and opportune treatment are especially important in the disease course as both can slow down or stop the disease from progressing to advanced stages, prevent complications, and reduce the number of associated cardiovascular events [6, 7].

Most people who reach end-stage kidney disease (ESKD) with renal replacement requirement are treated primarily with hemodialysis, peritoneal dialysis, and transplantation. The 5-year survival of people with CKD on dialysis is between 13% and 60% lower than people in the general population of similar ages [10].

Although dialysis therapy improves some symptoms and patient's survival, it does not cure the disease, has associated morbidity and mortality, and negatively affects the quality of life (QoL) of patients and their families. Moreover, it also has a high cost [6–8, 11–17].

In this context, finding treatment models that address all the needs of patients with ESKD who require opportune biopsychosocial and spiritual evaluations and optimizing the access to multidisciplinary health team are not only necessary but imperative. Accordingly, palliative medicine principles have been proposed as a model to comprehensively address the patient with ESKD [16–19].

C. Zuñiga-San Martin (✉)
Facultad de Medicina, Universidad Catolica de la Santisima Concepcion, Bio Bio, Chile

Facultad de Medicina, Universidad de Concepcion, Bio Bio, Chile

Instituto de Nefrologia Concepcion, Bio Bio, Chile

© Springer Nature Switzerland AG 2021

C. G. Musso et al. (eds.), *Frailty and Kidney Disease*,
https://doi.org/10.1007/978-3-030-53529-2_14

There is agreement in the nephrological community that renal conservative/palliative care improves symptoms and QoL in patients with CKD [18, 19]. In this chapter, we will review the relevance of including palliative care in nephrology and especially its role in comprehensive conservative care (non-dialytic treatment). This is an option for people with advanced CKD who, due to their deteriorated clinical condition or personal decision decide not to enter or to withdraw from dialysis therapy. Supportive and Conservative Care based on the principles of palliative medicine offers tremendous value not just to patients with CKD, families, and clinicians but also to all health system [18, 19].

Chronic Kidney Disease: Generalities

CKD is the alteration of renal function and/or structure produced by a heterogeneous group of diseases or conditions that affect different renal structures (glomerular, interstitial, or vascular compartment). Its evolution is generally irreversible and progressive in months or years toward the stage of advanced insufficiency where substitution therapies (dialysis or renal transplantation) are required [20].

The speed of progression is determined by multiple factors such as the cause of CKD, blood pressure control, proteinuria level, age, adherence and access to diagnosis and timely treatment, etc.

The main diseases that are susceptible and at high risk of developing CKD are diabetes mellitus, hypertension, obesity, and cardiovascular disease. It is well established that proper management and treatment of hypertension and diabetes mellitus are effective in slowing CKD progression and associated cardiovascular disease (CVD) risks, but unfortunately adverse outcomes for patients with CKD remain high.

The CKD diagnosis is made with at least one of the following criteria [8, 20]:

- Glomerular filtration rate (GFR) <60 mL/min/1.73 m^2. GFR can be estimated by serum creatinine level and GFR equations, such as MDRD-4 (Modification of Diet in Renal Disease) or CKD-EPI (Chronic Kidney Disease Epidemiology Collaboration).
- Renal damage is defined by the presence of:
  - Moderate/severe albuminuria (albumin/creatinine ratio (RAC) ≥30 mg/g)
  - Alterations of urine sediment, e.g., hematuria, blood cylinders
  - Electrolyte alterations or other alterations of tubular origin
  - Structural abnormalities (by ultrasound imaging, X-rays, magnetic resonance imaging)
  - Histological alterations (renal biopsy)
  - History of renal transplantation

CKD is classified into five stages [20] Table 14.1.

Table 14.1 CKD stages-KDIGO 2012 [20]

CKD STAGES- KDIGO 2012		
STAGES	**GFR (ml/min 1.73 m2)**	**DESCRPTION**
1	≥90	Kidney damage with normal or high GFR
2	60-89	Kidney damage with Mildly decreased GFR
3a	45-59	Mildly to moderately decreased
3b	30-44	Moderately to severely decreased
4	15-29	Severely decreased
5	<15	Kidney failure

In general, the current treatment of CKD is based on reducing noxas or conditions that cause damage to renal function and/or structure (diabetes mellitus, autoimmune diseases, vasculitis, glomerulopathies, among others) and, on the other hand, controling factors that induce progression (proteinuria, high blood pressure, hyperfiltration, acidosis, hyperuricemia, etc.).

In stage 5 of CKD, when kidney function is insufficient to conserving the vital requirements of the internal environment, the person affected by the disease must decide for one of the treatment options: renal replacement (hemo/peritoneal dialysis and renal transplantation) or comprehensive conservative care.

Frailty and Integrated ESKD Care

Renal Palliative Care

Palliative care was defined by the World Health Organization (WHO) as "comprehensive and interdisciplinary care, aimed at improving the QoL of the patient facing a life-threatening disease, through the prevention and relief of suffering" [17]. It includes the timely and adequate treatment of pain and other physical symptoms, along with the psychosocial and spiritual support of the patient and his family. In its definition, WHO considers the process of dying as a natural occurrence, affirms and promotes life, and does not intend to lengthen it unnecessarily or shorten it specifically, but to promote its quality. This perspective is applicable in any of the stages of the disease, from diagnosis until death [17].

Palliative care aims are:

- Support the patient and/or family with or at risk of developing a life-threatening (acute or chronic) condition:
  - Due to diagnosis
  - With any prognosis
  - Regardless of age
  - At any stage. Not only at the end of life
- Do not rush death or postpone it.
- Treat pain and associated symptoms (timely and adequate).
- Strengthen continuous care with multidisciplinary teams.
- Complement and potentiate curative therapy or work as a main treatment.

Why is palliative care applicable to patients with advanced CKD?

In patients with ESKD, physical and emotional symptoms are of high prevalence, and the number and intensity of symptoms is comparable to that reported by patients with cancer or AIDS [11–15]. Dialysis improves survival but not necessarily what the person considers quality of life. The comorbidities associated with CKD such as diabetes mellitus and cardiovascular disease are also progressive and contribute to the greater deterioration of the quality of life.

In addition, patients who access dialysis live the paradox of benefiting from these extraordinary advances in modern medicine and at the same time live their limitations. While dialysis helps them to sustain life by replacing nonfunctioning kidneys, the underlying systemic disease, such as diabetes mellitus, continues to progress, with neurological, motor sensory, visual, and QoL impairment. Dialysis therapy does not address the psychosocial, emotional, and spiritual aspects associated with the disease or treatment and the unfavorable impact on the QoL of people and their families.

Furthermore, the current profile of people entering dialysis has changed in recent years, with access to more older patients with two or three diseases associated with CKD such as diabetes mellitus, coronary heart disease, hypertension, heart failure, peripheral vascular disease, and cerebrovascular disease [1–6]. The current demographic trend of population aging and morbidity in many countries suggests that in the coming years, the number of geriatric patients with associated chronic and degenerative diseases will increase, as well as patients on dialysis treatment [1–6].

The progressive disability of patients with advanced CKD associated with the high burden of bio-psycho-emotional symptoms requires constant evaluation of their impact on QoL and timely interventions with multidisciplinary teams under the premises of the continuous palliative care model. The above requires a comprehensive therapeutic approach based on the incorporation of other professionals in the nephrology/dialysis units, such as social workers, psychologists, nutritionists, and kinesiologists, who support and contribute to the achievement of a better QoL for patients.

Considering the high burden of symptoms and psychosocial impact associated with the disease that affect people with CKD, it justifies the incorporation of a care model based on the principles of palliative medicine, whose main objective is to improve the QoL, in the comprehensive care of the renal patient, from diagnosis to advanced stages of the disease [15–19].

In cancer patients, supportive/palliative care has been traditionally applied in the last 6 months of life, because in that period the person suffers most of the ailments and aches associated to the disease. On the contrary, the QoL of patients with CKD is affected at an early stage, and its evolution is more heterogeneous and prolonged. Before reaching the ESRD, patients most frequently suffer from pain, asthenia, pruritus, dyspnea, anorexia, depressive symptoms, and insomnia [12–16]. Progressive disability and high burden of symptoms would require supportive/palliative care for a long time and usually long before the last year of life. In Table 14.2, you will find some support/palliative care issues closely related to nephrology and analysis, which have already been addressed in multiple specialty publications [16–19].

Which is the impact of quality of life on morbidity and mortality in CKD patients?

The published evidence indicates that there would be a close relationship between the QoL and the morbidity and mortality associated with the disease [21, 22]. Patients with CKD who report better QoL have fewer hospitalizations, lower morbidity and mortality, and greater adherence to treatment [21, 22]. Particularly, as we will see later, spirituality is an important component of the QoL construct, and therefore spiritual suffering would also affect clinical evolution [23] (Fig. 14.1).

Unfortunately, few people understand what renal palliative care is. Patients with CKD, family members, and the renal health team link the term "palliative care" with death, hospice, or end-of-life care, and some believe it should be offered only at the end of the disease, when there are no more dialysis therapies available.

Table 14.2 Palliative care topics in nephrology/dialysis

Pain management, sleep disorders, and sexual dysfunction associated with chronic kidney disease
Diagnosis and treatment of depression in dialysis
Ethical dilemmas associated with dialysis (not to start or withdrawal dialysis treatment)
Palliative care in pediatric nephrology and dialysis
Physical rehabilitation in dialysis
QoL evaluation in dialysis
Comprehensive conservative care of the renal patient at the end of life
Psychosocial and spiritual support to patients, family members, and caregivers
Self-care and QoL in health professionals

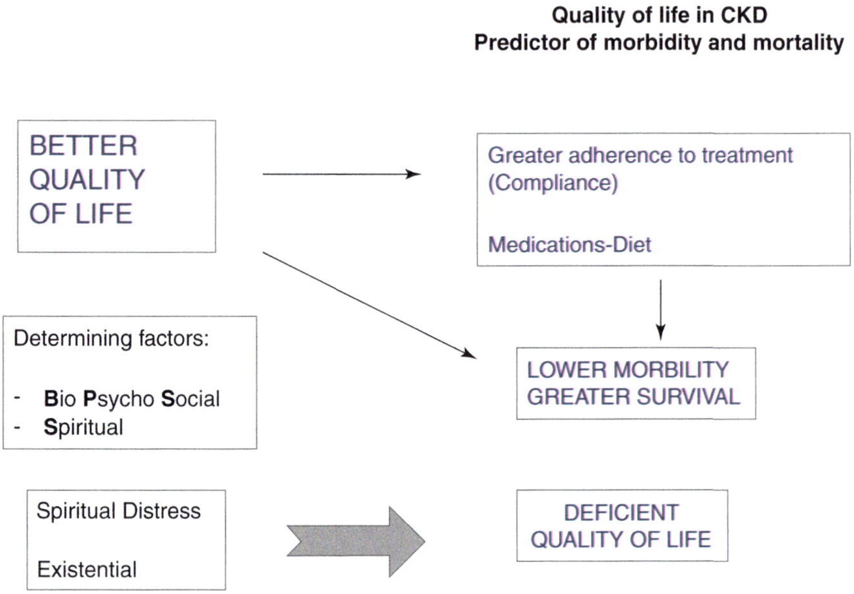

Fig. 14.1 Quality of life related to morbidity and mortality in advanced CKD patients

How care is currently being incorporated into the treatment of ESKD patients?

The current state of knowledge related to palliative care in advanced CKD patients, including those on dialysis, was agreed at the KDIGO Controversies Conference in 2012. An international group of multidisciplinary experts in CKD, palliative care, methodology, economics, and education identified the key issues related to palliative care in this population [18]. After that, in March 2018 the International Society of Nephrology (ISN) organized the 2nd Global Kidney Health Summit in United Arab Emirates. The purpose of the meeting was to develop a Integrated ESKD Care program to improve worldwide access to kidney replacement therapy (KRT) (i.e., dialysis or kidney transplantation) and non-KRT conservative care. A key component of treatment for all people with advanced kidney disease is supportive care, which aims to improve quality of life and can be provided alongside therapies intended to prolong life, such as dialysis. It incorporates the principles of palliative medicine in the care of patients with advanced CKD, promoting a comprehensive and continuous care [19].

What are Supportive care and Comprehensive Conservative care (Non-dialytic Treatment)?

Integrated ESKD Care program consider two intervention for the care of patients with advanced CKD: supportive care and comprehensive conservative care (Fig. 14.2).

A. *Supportive care* [18, 19, 24–26] involves services aimed at improving the QoL of patients with established CKD. It is based on the principles of palliative care, which is defined by the World Health Organization as an approach that improves

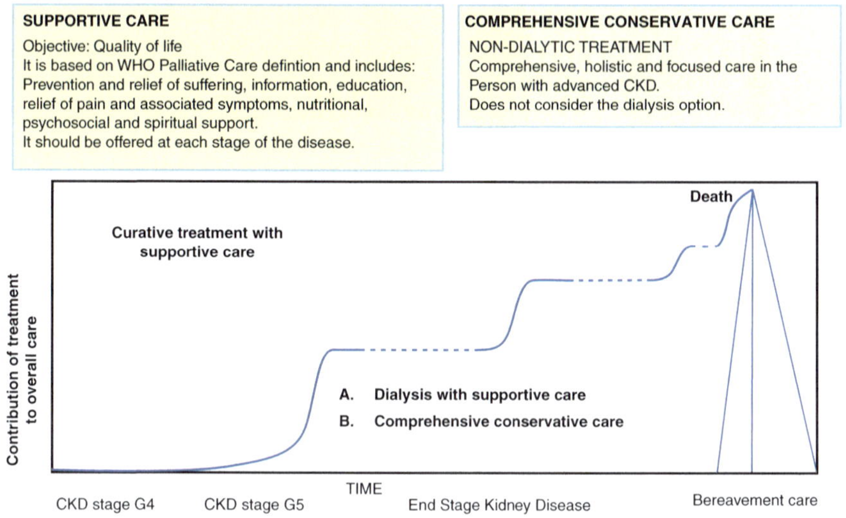

Fig. 14.2 An overview of the contribution of supportive and comprehensive conservative care to overall care in end stage kidney disease. Modified from Harris et al. [19]

the QoL of patients and their families facing problems associated with life-threatening illness, through the prevention and relief of suffering by means of early identification and impeccable assessment and treatment of pain and other physical, psychosocial, and spiritual problems. Supportive care should be offered at each stage of the disease, not only at the ESRD, including information, education, relief of pain and associated symptoms, nutritional support, and social and spiritual care.

B. *Comprehensive conservative care* [18, 19, 24–26] can be an alternative to renal replacement therapies (RRT). The comprehensive conservative care is where conservative care is either chosen or medically advised.

What is Comprehensive Conservative Care (Non-dialytic Treatment)

This is planned, holistic, person-centered care that includes the following:

- Interventions to delay progression of kidney disease and minimize risk of adverse events
- Shared decision-making
- Active symptom management
- Detailed communication including advance care planning
- Psychological support
- Social and family support
- Cultural and spiritual domains of care

Of note, comprehensive conservative care does not include dialysis.

It is important to emphasize that comprehensive conservative care (non-dialytic treatment) is an option that does not mean denying dialysis or less abandoning the patient. It is an option that has its own rules and indications.

Comprehensive conservative care is a new model of care for patients with advanced CKD that have emerged in different nephrology centers around the world. It is a new option considered as the fourth option after hemodialysis or peritoneal dialysis and transplant, and it is focused on comprehensive biopsychosocial care of the patient and his family [18–34].

This treatment option is indicated for patients with advanced CKD who also suffer from other disabling comorbidities, where dialysis therapy does not offer better QoL expectancy, or it is contraindicated and at risk due to a deteriorated and irreversible clinical condition [27–31]. Examples of disabling diseases with limited benefit of chronic dialysis treatment are presented in Table 14.3.

Conservative treatment incorporates the model of palliative medicine in renal patient care, based on the fact that the central objectives of this model are to improve the QoL through comprehensive care of the biopsychosocial aspects and affective/emotional and spiritual needs [24, 28, 29, 32].

Comprehensive conservative care does not replace dialysis when it is medically justified. It integrally addresses the patient with advanced CKD to optimize their QoL and alleviate the symptoms that limit it.

It is also an option for those patients and their legal representative who, once informed by the treatment team of the prognosis and the advantages/disadvantages of the different treatment options, express their willingness not to enter dialysis or to discontinue.

In practice, comprehensive conservative care consists of the monitoring and periodic evaluation by the multidisciplinary team and the application of medical and nutritional protocols and interventions aimed at halting or slowing progression to more advanced stages, as well as addressing the diagnosis and timely treatment of symptoms that impact QoL in the advanced stages of CKD [31–34].

It is fundamental for the achievement of the proposed objectives to carry out a cooperative, integrated, and coordinated work with the multidisciplinary teams composed of renal health teams, palliativists, geriatricians, nutritionists, psychologists, social workers, physiatrists, and spiritual support [33, 34]. This will allow offering the best available options, especially in the stage of prostration and home care of patients who chose not to start or discontinue a dialysis therapy [27, 30, 31].

Table 14.3 Invaliding diseases with limited benefit with chronic dialysis

Neurological diseases with severe and irreversible cognitive and motor sequelae
Advanced heart failure associated with myocardial infarction
Terminal renal disease not caused beyond therapeutic range
Older patient in a condition of irreversible fragility
Advanced dementia or severe psychiatric disorder (a condition that contraindicates and/or increases the risk of the dialysis procedure)

What Does It Include and Where It Is Done?

In the absence of resource constraints, Integrated ESKD care should ideally be available as an integrated mix of peritoneal/haemodialysis, transplantation, and comprehensive conservative care (non-dialytic treatment), and patients should be able to choose and transition between the different modalities [9]. The first step is the evaluation of the patient by the multidisciplinary team and then the options are offered and requests the corresponding informed consent to the patien and/or his legal representative.

In practice, the comprehensive conservative care consists of monitoring and periodic evaluation (monthly or bimonthly) by the multidisciplinary team and the application of medical protocols and interventions for the timely treatment of symptoms that impact the QoL in the advanced stages of CKD. It includes pain management, sleep disorders, depression, sexual dysfunction, containment, and psychosocial and spiritual support for patients and families.

This treatment option must be delivered in units attached to those of dialysis or nephrology since it is a therapeutic option that is offered to those patients with advanced CKD and therefore must be addressed by the nephrological health team [34].

What Role Does the Spiritual Dimension Play in the Integral Care of Patients with Advanced CKD?

It is recognized that CKD imposes intense physical and psychosocial stress on the patient that defies his sense of life, his vision, and his expectation of the future. Occasionally, the spiritual/religious practice becomes the main pillar of support that the patient has to face and make sense of the suffering associated with the disease and treatment.

In this regard, there are already reports that study in patients with advanced CKD the spiritual/religious aspects of the patient and their association with QoL, psychosocial impact, and adherence to treatment, which would be influenced independently of the biomedical aspects of the disease and/or the type of treatment [35–41]. This dimension of the human being has been included in the definition of palliative care of the WHO and in the ISN Integrated ESKD Care program [18, 19].

The QoL is a construct, based on the perception of the person and the assessment assigned to their physical, emotional, functional, social, and spiritual well-being, after diagnosis and treatment. Considering that the spiritual/religious or existential dimension is one of the pillars of the definition, its evaluation and impact on the QoL of the chronic renal patient acquires relevance [23, 35–41] (Fig. 14.1).

Table 14.4 Frequently asked questions or comments from patients would suggest need for support in the spiritual dimension

Why did this chronic kidney disease occur to me?
What is the meaning of suffering in this life connected to a dialysis machine?
What fault am I paying?
What did I do wrong to make this happen to me?
Has my life really been worth it?
If I die, who will take care of my loved ones?
If there is a God, why do you punish me with this suffering from dialysis?
Is there another life after this?
How can I relax and have peace on dialysis?

It has been reported in dialysis patients that spiritual well-being is associated with better quality and satisfaction of life, strengthens family/social support, decreases depressive symptomatology, generates greater adherence to treatment, and is associated with fewer hospitalizations and lower morbidity and mortality. On the contrary, a spiritual distress entails a poor QoL and negatively impacts evolution and medical outcomes [23, 35–41] (Fig. 14.1).

The manifestations of distress or spiritual suffering demonstrate itself in various ways. In particular, patients manifest hopelessness, absence of existential sense, or feelings of worthlessness and devaluation [23, 41].

Patients with advanced CKD have spiritual/existential needs that are usually not investigated and also not addressed. These needs would be independent of the age, time, and type of disease.

There are no predictors to anticipate those who provide spiritual support, and some questions or comments from patients with CKD described in Table 14.4 could be an alert of the need for support in the spiritual dimension [41]. Medical teams should familiarize themselves with them so that it is necessary to make a timely referral and/or intervention by professionals in charge of spiritual support and accompaniment. The extension and nature of the spiritual and existential issues thus validates the need to diversify the composition of the multidisciplinary teams for a comprehensive care of patients with advanced CKD.

The renal health teams might consider that addressing spiritual needs does not correspond to their competence, let alone solve such complex existential questions of the human being. However, this does not exempt them from maintaining a compassionate attitude toward their patient and being present, close, and available to recognize the spiritual/existential needs that could cause psychosocial distress and affect the acceptance of the disease and/or adaptation to treatment [23, 41]. This attitude, in addition to improving the medical team/patient relationship, allows other professionals with more experience to provide support in this area (psychologists, social workers, spiritual companions, etc.) when it is considered appropriate and in consensus with the patient.

The regular practice of activities related to spirituality/religiosity in patients with advanced CKD would be positively associated with better QoL, satisfaction with medical care, and psychosocial support [23, 35–41].

Also, the spiritual/existential well-being would contribute to the mental health of the person by attenuating the depressive and anxious symptoms that patients on dialysis frequently manifest. It also constitutes an important source of comfort and hope that strengthens and is synergistic with the support provided by family and social support networks [23–41]. These benefits would be independent of the age, comorbidities, and time of the disease.

Moreover, in the advanced stages of the disease and especially at the end of life, addressing the spiritual/religious or existential dimension could be as or more important than physical well-being, and it is imperative to consider in the planning of comprehensive care.

Spirituality is inherent in our human condition and therefore always needs to be assessed its level of well-being and intervene in a timely manner when required if we wish to grant comprehensive care and improve the QoL of our patients with advanced CKD.

Ethical Considerations in the Decision to Enter or Not to Dialysis

The progressive increase in patients admitted to renal replacement therapies (RRT) raises multiple ethical challenges. Health teams must participate in the decision to enter, maintain, or suspend dialysis to patients in whom, due to their precarious state of mental health, multiple comorbidities, or poor QoL expectancy, it is not expected to obtain a greater benefit with the renal replacement therapies (RRT) [42–48]. Dialytic therapies like any medical treatment have indications and contraindications; therefore, the decision to enter or not, as well as when to start them or which one to use, should result from an informed and agreed choice between the patient, his medical team, and the family, opting for the best therapeutic alternative, including conservative management [18, 19, 42–48]. It should always be kept in mind that RRTs can prolong life but not necessarily their quality and that not all patients benefit from them.

Elderly people with multiple comorbidities, frailty, or important functional sequelae are those who most raise ethical challenges related to the decision to enter or leave dialysis [42–47]. An ethical challenge thus arises: whether or not to enter dialysis for patients with these characteristics? The question is justified by comparing the evolution and survival with those patients who, under the same limited clinical conditions, choose to receive only conservative treatment and not enter chronic dialysis [18, 19, 27–32, 43–47]. In these people, the dialysis does not improve the symptomatology, and on the contrary many times it accentuates the disabling symptoms, it deteriorates more its fragility, QoL and for some it does not even imply greater survival. The advantage of dialysis under these conditions would be substantially reduced by disabling comorbidities, and the option of conservative treatment would obtain equal survival and a better QoL for the patient and the family. Choosing to enter or not dialysis, as well as when to start or which one to use, should always result from an informed and consensual choice between the patient, his medical team, and the family, include the option of comprehensive conservative care (non-dialytic treatment) [18, 19, 43–47]. In this regard, it has been proposed to reconsider some criteria for admission to dialysis, based on multiple studies where it has been shown that elderly and fragile patients with a high number of disabling comorbidities obtain minimal benefits with dialysis treatment and for some it does not even imply greater survival [44–48]. (See Table 14.3: Diseases with limited benefit of chronic dialysis.). The added value that implies the timely and adequate delivery of information so in consensus with the patient and his family to opt for the best treatment is to guarantee due respect and consideration of the ethical principles of autonomy, beneficence, non-maleficence, and justice that are accepted as substantial in medical practice.

In summary, there is evidence that the QoL of patients with CKD especially in the advanced stages is affected by the high burden of physical symptoms and psychosocial changes that negatively impact their lives and that of their families. Usually, patients report pain, asthenia, pruritus, dyspnea, anorexia, depressive symptoms, and insomnia with variable intensity and frequency. About it, the International Society of Nephrology proposed in 2018 a Integrated ESKD Care program. Based on the principles of palliative medicine and participation of multidisciplinary teams, it recommends a continuous and integral biopsychosocial and spiritual care of patients with CKD and includes support in the grieving process for family members. It includes the supportive care that comprehensively addresses the patient with established CKD to optimize their QoL and relieve the symptoms that limit it in any of its stages, with or without dialysis. It also incorporates comprehensive conservative care (non-dialytic conservative treatment) as another treatment option along with hemodialysis, peritoneal dialysis, and renal transplantation [18, 19]. Comprehensive conservative care is especially aimed at patients with advanced CKD who also suffer from other disabling comorbidities, where dialysis therapy does not offer better quality of life expectancy or is contraindicated and is at risk due to a deteriorated and irreversible clinical condition. They are continuous palliative support care focused on the sick person and their family. It is also an option for those patients and their legal representative who freely, once informed by the prognosis team of the advantages/disadvantages of the different treatment options, express their willingness not to enter dialysis or discontinue if the patient is already using it [43, 46–48].

References

1. Hill NR, Fatoba ST, Oke JL, Hirst JA, O'Callaghan CA, Lasserson DS, Hobbs FDR. Global prevalence of chronic kidney disease – a systematic review and meta-analysis. PLoS One. 2016;11(7):e0158765.
2. Neuen BL, Chadban SJ, Demaio AR, Johnson DW, Perkovic V. Chronic kidney disease and the global NCDs agenda. BMJ Glob Health. 2017;2(2):e000380.
3. GBD Collaborators. Mortality GBD, Causes of Death C. Global, regional, and national age-sex specific all-cause and cause-specific mortality for 240 causes of death, 1990–2013: a systematic analysis for the Global Burden of Disease Study 2013. Lancet. 2015;385(9963):117–71.

4. GBD Collaborators. Global, regional, and national incidence, prevalence, and years lived with disability for 301 acute and chronic diseases and injuries in 188 countries, 1990–2013: a systematic analysis for the Global Burden of Disease Study 2013. Lancet. 2015;386(9995):743–800.
5. Poblete H. Chilean nephrology society. Dialysis register 2018. Last access, 15 July 2019. Available at: https://www.nefro.cl/v2/biblio/registro/24.pdf.
6. Eckardt KU, Coresh J, Devuyst O, Johnson RJ, Kottgen A, Levey AS, et al. Evolving importance of kidney disease: from subspecialty to global health burden. Lancet. 2013;382(9887):158–69.
7. Go AS, Chertow GM, Fan D, McCulloch CE, Hsu CY. Chronic kidney disease and the risks of death, cardiovascular events, and hospitalization. N Engl J Med. 2004;351(13):1296–305.
8. Stevens PE, Levin A, Kidney Disease: Improving Global Outcomes Chronic Kidney Disease Guideline Development Work Group Members. Evaluation and management of chronic kidney disease: synopsis of the kidney disease: improving global outcomes 2012 clinical practice guideline. Ann Intern Med. 2013;158(11):825–30.
9. Institute for Health Metrics and Evaluation [Internet]. [cited 2018 Mar 15]. Available from: http://www.healthdata.org/.
10. Webster AC, Nagler EV, Morton RL, Masson P. Chronic kidney disease. Lancet. 2017;389(10075):1238–52. Available from: http://www.ncbi.nlm.nih.gov/pubmed/27887750
11. Kalantar- Kalantar-Zadeh K, Kopple JD, Block G, Humphreys MH. Association among SF36 quality of life measures and nutrition, hospitalization and mortality in haemodialysis. J Am Soc Nephrol. 2001;12:2797–806.
12. Zuniga C, Dapueto J, Müller H, Kirsten L, Alid R, Ortiz L. Health related quality of life among patients on chronic haemodialysis. Rev Med Chile. 2009;137:200–7.
13. Weisbord SD, Fried LF, Arnold RM, Fine MJ, Levenson DJ, Peterson RA, et al. Prevalence, severity, and importance of physical and emotional symptoms in chronic hemodialysis patients. J Am Soc Nephrol. 2005;16:2487–94.
14. Murtagh FE, Addington-Hall J, Higginson IJ. The prevalence of symptoms in end-stage renal disease: a systematic review. Adv Chronic Kidney Dis. 2007;14:82–99.
15. Weisbord SD, Carmody SS, Bruns FJ, Rotondi AJ, Cohen LM, Zeidel ML, et al. Symptom burden, quality of life, advance care planning and the potential value of palliative care in severely ill haemodialysis patients. Nephrol Dial Transplant. 2003;18:1345–52.
16. Germain MJ, Kurella Tamura M, Davison SN. Palliative care in CKD: the earlier the better. Am J Kidney Dis. 2011;57(3):378–80.
17. World Health Organization. WHO definition of palliative care. Available at: http://www.who.int/cancer/palliative/definition/en/. Accessed 5 Apr 2018.
18. Davison SN, Levin A, Moss AH, et al. Executive summary of the KDIGO Controversies Conference on Supportive Care in Chronic Kidney Disease: developing a roadmap to improving quality care. Kidney Int. 2015;88(3):447–59.
19. Harris DCH, Davies SJ, Finkelstein FO, Jha V, Donner JA, et al. Increasing access to integrated ESKD care as part of universal health coverage. Kidney Int. 2019;95(4 Suppl):S1–S33.
20. Levey AS, Eckardt KU, Tsukamoto Y, Levin A, Coresh J, Rossert J, et al. Definition and classification of chronic kidney disease: a position statement from Kidney Disease: Improving Global Outcomes (KDIGO). Kidney Int. 2005;67(6):2089–100.
21. Finkelstein FO, Wuerth D, Finkelstein SH. Health related quality of life and the CKD patient: challenges for the nephrology community. Kidney Int. 2009;76:946–52.
22. Mapes DL, Lopes AA, Satayathum SS, Mccullough KP, Goodkin DA, Locatelli F, et al. Health-related quality of life as a predictor of mortality and hospitalization: the Dialysis outcome and practice pattern study (DOPPS). Kidney Int. 2003;64(1):339–49.
23. Davison SN, Jhangri GS. The relationship between spirituality, psychosocial adjustment to illness, and health-related quality of life in patients with advanced chronic kidney disease. J Pain Symptom Manag. 2013;45:170–8.
24. Harris DCH, Davies SJ, Finkelstein FO, Jha V. The second Global Kidney Health Summit outputs: developing a strategic plan to increase access to integrated end-stage kidney disease care worldwide. Kidney Int Suppl. 2020;10(1):e1–e2.

25. Swanepoel CR, McCulloch MI, Abraham G, Donner JA, Alrukhaimi MN, Blake PG, Bunnag S, et al. Challenges for sustainable end-stage kidney disease care in low-middle-income countries: the problem of the workforce. Kidney Int Suppl. 2020;10:e49–e54.
26. Hole B, Hemmelgarn B, Brown E, Brown M, McCulloch MI, Zuniga C, et al. Supportive care for end-stage kidney disease: an integral part of kidney services across a range of income settings around the world. Kidney Int Suppl. 2020;10:e86–e94.
27. Hussain JA, Mooney A, Russon L. Comparison of survival analysis and palliative care involvement in patients aged over 70 years choosing conservative management or renal replacement therapy in advanced chronic kidney disease. Palliat Med. 2013;27(9):829–39.
28. Alston H, Burns A. Conservative care of the patient with end-stage renal disease. Clin Med. 2015;15(6):567–70.
29. O'Connor NR, Kumar P. Conservative management of end-stage renal disease without dialysis: a systematic review. J Palliat Med. 2012;15(2):228–35.
30. Song MK. Quality of life of patients with advanced chronic kidney disease receiving conservative care without Dialysis. Semin Dial. 2016;29(2):165–9.
31. Raghavan D, Holley JL. Conservative care of the elderly CKD patient: a practical guide. Adv Chronic Kidney Dis. 2016;23(1):51–6.
32. Dattolo P, Michelassi S, Amidone M, Allinovi M, Vignali L, Antognoli G, et al. Structured clinical follow-up for CKD stage 5 may safely postpone dialysis. J Nephrol. 2015;28(4):463–9.
33. Chen PM, Lai TS, Chen PY, Lai CF, Yang SY, Wu V, et al. Multidisciplinary care program for advanced chronic kidney disease: reduces renal replacement and medical costs. Am J Med. 2015;128(1):68–76.
34. Zuniga C. Support/palliative care. Why, when and how? Dial Traspl. 2014;35(1):20–6.
35. Finkelstein SH, West W, Gobin J, Finkelstein SH, Wuerth D. Spirituality, quality of life and the dialysis patient. Nephrol Dial Transplant. 2007;22:2432–4.
36. Kimmel PL, Emont SL, Newmann JM, Danko H, Moss AH. ESRD patient quality of life symptoms, spiritual beliefs, psychosocial factors. Am J Kidney Dis. 2003;42:713–21.
37. Lucchetti G, de Almeida LGC, Lucchetti ALG. Religiousness, mental health, and quality of life in Brazilian dialysis patients. Hemodial Int. 2012;16:89–94.
38. Saffari ML, Pakpour AH, Naderi MK, Koenig HG, Baldacchino DR, Piper CN. Spiritual coping, religiosity and quality of life a study on Muslim patients undergoing haemodialysis. Nephrology (Carlton). 2013;18:269–75.
39. Al-Ghabeesh SH, Alshraifeen AA, Saifan AR, Bashayreh IH, Alnuaimi KM, Masalha HA. Spirituality in the lives of patients with end-stage renal disease: a systematic review. J Relig Health. 2018;57:2461–77.
40. Spinale J, Cohen SD, Khetpal P, Peterson RA, Clougherty B, Puchalski C, et al. Spirituality, social support, and survival in hemodialysis patients. Clin J Am Soc Nephrol. 2008;3(6):1620–7.
41. Davison SN, Jhangri GS. Existential and supportive care needs among patients with chronic kidney disease. J Pain Symptom Manag. 2010;40(6):838–43.
42. Moss AH. Revised dialysis clinical practice guideline promotes more informed decision-making. Clin J Am Soc Nephrol. 2010;5:2380.
43. Moss AH. Ethical principles and processes guiding dialysis, decision-making. Clin J Am Soc Nephrol. 2011;6:2313.
44. Singh P, Germain MJ, Cohen L, Unruh M. The elderly patient on dialysis: geriatric considerations. Nephrol Dial Transplant. 2014;29(5):990–6.
45. Johansen KL, Chertow GM, Jin C, Kutner NG. Significance of frailty among dialysis patients. J Am Soc Nephrol. 2007;18:2960–7.
46. White Y, Fitzpatrick G. *Dialysis*: prolonging life or prolonging dying? Ethical, legal and professional considerations for end of life decision making. EDTNA ERCA J. 2006;32(2):99–103.
47. Germain MJ, Davison SN, Moss AH. When enough is enough: the nephrologist's responsibility in ordering dialysis treatments. Am J Kidney Dis. 2011;58(1):135–43.
48. Germain MJ, Cohen LM, Davison SN. Withholding and withdrawal from dialysis: what we know about how our patients die. Semin Dial. 2007;20(3):195–9.

Index

© Springer Nature Switzerland AG 2021

C. G. Musso et al. (eds.), *Frailty and Kidney Disease*,
https://doi.org/10.1007/978-3-030-53529-2

9783030535285